AN EASY GUIDE TO AYURVEDA

AN EASY GUIDE TO
AYURVEDA
THE NATURAL WAY TO WHOLENESS

*Basic Principles,
Practices, and Routines
for Total Well-Being,
Rapid Spiritual Growth,
and Effective Living*

ROY EUGENE DAVIS

CSA PRESS, *PUBLISHERS*
CENTER FOR SPIRITUAL AWARENESS
Lakemont, Georgia 30552

CSA Press, Publishers
Lake Rabun Road, P.O. Box 7
Lakemont, Georgia 30552 (U.S.A.)
Telephone (706) 782-4723
Fax (706) 782-4560

. . CSA Press is the publishing department
of Center for Spiritual Awareness, with offices
and retreat center on Lake Rabun Road.

In West Africa:
Centre for Spiritual Awareness
Post Office Box 507, Accra, Ghana

For addresses of distributors in other regions
of the world, contact the publisher.

PHOTOS:
Ryan Hooper and Kathleen Low

Printed and manufactured in the United States of America

INTRODUCTION

In the following pages I have explained fundamental principles, practices, and lifestyle routines of Ayurveda (*I´-yur-vāde-a*, life-knowledge), a natural system for health and actualization of spiritual potential.

Because of a growing interest in health self-care, information about Ayurvedic regimens and products is increasingly appearing in the secular media and in specialized publications. A word to the wise: The ideal teacher or practitioner of Ayurveda is one who is well-grounded in the philosophy and principles and who lives accordingly. Advertised products should not be used unless with qualified advice or accurate, self-trained knowledge. Foods and herbal compounds should be chosen for their known benefits and absence of unwanted side effects. When considering advice or products, always carefully determine the quality of the source.

Within the past few decades, because of an increasing willingness of people the world over to be self-responsible for their lives, Ayurvedic procedures have been beneficially adopted in many regions of the world. Because our well-being is intimately related to our self-chosen behaviors, the guidelines described here will be helpful to the extent that they are thoughtfully and appropriately applied.

I am not suggesting that readers being helped by their physician or health care provider discontinue that relationship in favor of exclusive self-treatment. While we need to be responsible for our wellness, we also need to use common sense when the knowledge and services of qualified care-givers are necessary.

Some of the information presented here was first published as a series of monthly lessons distributed to our members in North America and several countries. I have revised parts of the original text and added much new information to make the overall presentation more comprehensive and helpful. In some instances, Sanskrit word definitions are provided. Having an intellectual grasp of the meanings of the Sanskrit words can be helpful in acquiring intuitive insight into the full scope of the philosophical basis of the Ayurvedic approach to restoring and maintaining Spirit-mind-body balance, which is the purpose of the recommended practices and routines.

To improve health and function only for the purpose of continuing a self-centered, sense-oriented life is of minimal value. The ideal approach to life-enhancement is one which enables us to actualize healthy, long life and to accomplish constructive purposes.

ROY EUGENE DAVIS

Lakemont, Georgia (U.S.A.)
Summer, 1996

Contents

1

Basic Principles, Practices, and Lifestyle Routines for Total Wellness

Ayurveda evolved in India more than two thousand years ago. Because this knowledge is believed to have emerged into human consciousness from the Infinite Field of Being which is the common reality of all souls, it is said that it was taught to people by the gods. It spread eastward throughout Asia, and westward via the Mediterranean countries and Europe. During British rule in India, Ayurvedic practices declined in the urban centers while remaining the treatment of choice among rural populations. There are several Ayurvedic colleges in India, and schools and clinics are rapidly becoming available in Europe and America as public awareness increases and more people are seeking ways to help themselves to actualize and maintain total wellness. The two major Ayurvedic texts are *Charaka Samhita* and *Sushruta Samhita*. Charaka and Sushruta are the names of the compilers of the *samhitas*, the collected information.

Diagnostic procedures include examination of the pulse, body temperature, skin, eyes, tongue, urine, physiological systems, observed and reported behaviors, psychological characteristics, and other factors which might reveal the causes of discomfort and provide insight into determining the precise therapeutic regimen needed to restore balanced wholeness.

Ayurvedic practitioners are fond of quoting the axiom:

"One should be more interested in what kind of patient has the symptoms than in what kind of symptoms the patient has." While knowledge of symptoms is necessary, of primary importance is to know the basic mind-body constitution of the person being examined. When the body-mind constitution is restored to balance, optimum psychological and physical health can be established and maintained.

When there is habitual spiritual, mental, emotional, or physical imbalance, or persistent, disturbed personal or environmental circumstances, healing is needed. Treatment may include spiritual practices, psychological evaluation, necessary adjustments of mental attitudes and thinking habits, regulation of emotional states, behavior modification, body cleansing procedures, exercise, rest, foods to provide nutrition as well as for psychological and physical balance, ideal environment, cheerful and supportive personal relationships, herbs, colors, gems, metals, and whatever else might be nurturing and life-enhancing. The aim is not merely to suppress symptoms of discomfort or disease; it is to remove underlying causes so that healing is complete and permanent.

Right Living Contributes to Healthy, Long Life with Enlightened Purpose

We are not in this world only to survive and consume natural resources; we are here to live skillfully and freely with enlightened (clearly known) purpose. For this, four soul urges have to be fulfilled:

- To live in harmony with nature so that we have its full support and it has ours.
- To have our life-enhancing desires easily fulfilled to effectively accomplish our purposes.
- To be freely functional and receptive to life and have needs spontaneously met without strain.
- To experience authentic spiritual growth that results in illumination of mind and consciousness.

For anyone intent upon illumination of consciousness and unrestricted living, there are specific regimens and practices for vitalizing the body, energizing the mind, and clearing awareness so that necessary knowledge can be acquired and Self-revealed.

To experience immediate benefits, it is not necessary at the outset that the reasons for the effectiveness of these procedures be fully understood. They are based on natural laws—the principles of causation which determine processes occurring in the universe—and results will be in accord with their appropriate application. With added learning and right application, understanding will improve and intuitive knowledge of the causative principles inherent in life's processes will be acquired.

Do not limit yourself by thinking that it is difficult to live effectively. Allow yourself time to learn and to experience the results of applying what you learn. If some of the fundamental concepts are different from what you have heard or believed until now, be reassured by the fact that, as insight dawns, the principles supporting this practical approach to wellness will be comprehended.

Sequence of Cosmic Manifestation

Field of Absolute Pure Consciousness
|
Emanation of Consciousness Because of Impulse to Express
Field of God: Consciousness—Existence—Creative Power.
|
Om
|
Om Manifesting as Primordial Nature (*Maya*)
Energy of Om, time, space, and essences of cosmic particles
influenced by the gunas: sattva, rajas, tamas.
|
Field of Cosmic Mind
|
Eight Aspects of Intelligence of Consciousness in Om
Particularized and pervasive at causal, astral, and physical levels
influential in manifestation, preservation, and dissolution; as All
Pervading Consciousness; and as Reflected Consciousness.
|
Individualization of Consciousness (*Atman*)
Self-Awareness and Ego—the false sense of independent existence.
|
Intelligence (*Buddhi*) and Individualized Mind (*Manas*)
|
Subtle Organs of Sense Perception (*Jnanendriyas*)
Hearing   Touch   Sight   Taste   Smell
|
Subtle Organs of Actions (*Karmendriyas*)
Speech   Walking   Manual Dexterity   Elimination   Reproduction
|
Sense Objects (*Tanmatras*)
Ether   Air   Fire   Water   Earth

The Origins, Actions, and Influences of Nature's Three Influential Principles

Everything in nature has origins in the unmodified Field of Absolute Pure Consciousness. From this realm, the first emanation that expands into manifestation is Consciousness with attributes of Being, Awareness, and Power—that which is commonly referred to as God. From God, a flow of creative force (Om) manifests with four aspects: as a vibrational frequency; particles with potential to manifest matter; space; and time. This is the field or realm of primordial nature, the substance of which the universe and our bodies are comprised.

Our origin is also the Field of Absolute Pure Consciousness. In truth, Consciousness is what we are. The radiance of God's light shining on the field of primordial nature reflects as individualized rays or units of God's consciousness. When individualized rays or units of God's consciousness further identify with mind and matter, they are referred to as souls. Souls only identify with or relate to mind and matter; they do not become mind or matter.

The essence of every soul, the true Self of us, is ever individualized Pure Consciousness. It is important that we remember this because it means that we are spiritual beings expressing through a mind and body. We are, therefore, other than, and superior to, mind and body. This is why we should never think, believe, feel, or behave as though we are helpless effects of mental or material conditions or circumstances.

If we are in need of healing or of having improved circumstances of any kind, it is helpful to view ourselves in the right perspective in relationship to our thoughts, feelings, behaviors, and circumstances. We can then make right choices and implement constructive actions to effect desired transformations and changes. If we forget that we have the ability to cause effects, or refuse to use (or unwisely use) the knowledge we have, we put ourselves in a relationship with life which causes us to be victims of circumstances. Improvement is then difficult to experience because our spiritual potential is restricted.

Even with an advanced degree of knowledge of how to live, if we are not established in right Self-understanding, we may consciously endeavor to do everything supportive of our desire to experience improvement while unconsciously interfering with our return to wholeness by clinging to the delusion (intellectual error) that we are helpless, or that our well-being is entirely dependent upon external influences. Even so, if we do constructive things, some benefit will result which may assist us to degrees of wellness which enable us to understand more fully our spiritual nature and the basic principles of causation.

The three influential principles which regulate and govern environmental and biological processes emanate from the field of primordial nature and pervade the universe. They are qualities of cosmic forces with attributes. The Sanskrit word used to designate them is *guna* (an influence that regulates cosmic forces). *Sattva* (*sat*, is-ness, truth, being) *guna* is the force of equilibrium expressive as goodness, purity, harmony, balance, happiness, virtue, and knowledge. *Rajas* (*raj*, to glow, to be dynamically active) *guna* is the force of energy and motion expressive as passion, action, contention, and desire. *Tamas* (*tam*, to decline or perish) *guna* is the force of inaction, darkness, inertia, and obscurity.

Sattva guna contributes to mental illumination, general well-being, easy ability to appropriately adapt to circumstances, clarity of purpose, appreciation of order, refinement of the body and personality, and progressive spiritual growth.

Rajas guna contributes to goal-oriented endeavor, resistance to contrary conditions, attempts to dominate, assertion of will, and inclination to create and aspire.

Tamas guna contributes to clouded mental faculties, confusion, delusion (false or invalid beliefs and opinions), illusion (misperception), emotional heaviness, laziness, dullness, indifference to change and new experiences, and unconsciousness. It opposes the influences of both *sattva guna* and *rajas guna*.

All of the qualities of nature somewhat restrict the soul's expression because of their tendency to exert influence. *Tamas* restricts through negligence, errors of perception and behavior, and inaction, thus suppressing knowledge and contributing to the false sense of independent consciousness. *Rajas* encourages vanity and egocentric ambition, strong desire, perverted behaviors, and attachments and aversions. *Sattva* restricts because even though one may be motivated by idealism, self-conscious inclinations toward acquiring virtue and knowledge as ends in themselves may prevail.

We are well-advised to work with the *gunas*: transforming the heaviness of *tamas* by constructive, *rajasic* actions and behaviors as inspired by illuminating *sattvic* influences until soul knowledge and spontaneous inclinations to live correctly become determining factors.

A field of Universal Mind is produced from the field of primordial nature which, because of the actions of the

Field of Absolute, Unmanifest Pure Consciousness

Manifest Consciousness: God

Primordial Nature
Om, Cosmic Particles, Space, Time

Universal Mind-Substance

Influential Attributes (Gunas)

Sattva   Rajas   Tamas

Ether   Air   Fire   Water   Earth

Vata Dosha   Pitta Dosha   Kapha Dosha
The governing principles of biological functions.

Six Tastes Derived From Primary Element Influences

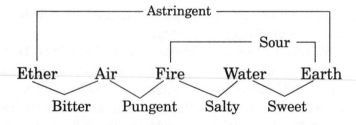

The tastes of the element influences increase the doshas with corresponding origins. The other tastes decrease them.

gunas, produces five fine, primary element influences of ether (space with cosmic particles with potential to express or manifest), air, fire, water, and earth, which can manifest in physical form as space, gaseous substances, radiance, moisture, and cohesive matter. The ether element is produced from *sattva guna*. The air element is produced from *sattva* and *rajas*. The fire element is produced from *rajas guna*. The water element is produced from *rajas* and *tamas*. The earth element is produced from *tamas guna*. The influences of all three *gunas* are present when dominant ones are obvious.

The *gunas*, through the element-influences, express as governing principles (*doshas*) which regulate nature's processes. From the combined influences of ether and air, the air principle (*vata dosha*) manifests. From the combined actions of fire and water influences, the fire principle (*pitta dosha*) manifests. *Kapha dosha* manifests from water and earth influences.

Vata dosha governs movement and circulation in nature and in living things. *Pitta dosha* governs metabolism, temperature, eyesight, and mental alertness. *Kapha dosha* is the moistening and lubricating influence. These descriptions are brief; a more complete examination of the *doshas* and their influences will be made as we progress with our study. When the three governing principles are balanced, psychological and physical health is the normal state. When one or more are disturbed, or are excessive or deficient, discomfort and sometimes disease can occur. Ayurvedic regimens and practices are chosen to restore the *doshas* to a harmonious relationship.

A Practical, Experimental Application of Routines and Practices for Overall Wellness

The best way to experience the life-enhancing benefits of this natural approach to wholeness is to enter into an experimental and experiential program. All of the routines and practices recommended are life-enhancing because their implementation contributes to orderly circumstances and total wellness.

To begin, use the chart provided at the end of this chapter to determine your basic psychophysiological (mind-body) constitution. Doing this will enable you to better relate to the information provided in this book, as well as provide knowledge of yourself and how what you do (and what occurs around you) might influence your awareness, mind, body, and circumstances.

The basic mind-body constitution of your parents, the prevailing circumstances experienced by your mother during the months before you were born, the characteristics you brought with you to this realm, and subtle environmental influences present at your physical birth, were determining factors in providing you with your basic mind-body constitution, which does not change. Many factors past and present have also influenced your basic constitution. If you were born with a balanced constitution and have lived a healthy, stress-free life, you are probably healthy, functional, and happy. If your constitution was sound but your lifestyle has been unhealthy and stress and trauma have been common, you may presently have some challenges to overcome or situations to improve. If you have always been unwell, restoration to wholeness is needed. Whatever your present state of spiritual, mental, emotional, or circumstantial health, an intentional, natural lifestyle will be supportive of total wellness and more effective living. The following practices can be included in daily routines:

- Go to sleep before 10 p.m. and awaken before sunrise. You will sleep better, and the early morning influences will help you begin your day with optimism and an awareness of real purpose.
- Attend to bathroom routines.
- Pray and meditate. Do this for at least 20 minutes, longer if you prefer. Your meditation session may be preceded by gentle hatha yoga practice or simple stretching exercises—this is optional.
- Have a light breakfast. *Kapha* constitutional types may wait until 10 a.m. or later to eat the first light meal of the day.
- Wear clean, comfortable clothing.
- Begin your work or activities for the day.
- Have your main meal between noon and 2 p.m. For all meals, choose natural foods agreeable to your mind-body constitution. Have all six tastes (sweet, sour, salty, pungent, astringent, and bitter) included at your main meal; more of the tastes helpful to maintaining *doshic* balance and less of the others. Have meals in a quiet, pleasant environment. Rest for a few minutes after eating, or take a short, relaxed walk. (Food tastes and their influences are explained in chapter 3.)
- Continue work or activities.
- Late afternoon or early evening, meditate, and relax.
- Have a light evening meal. Rest or go for a short walk. Meditate again if you want to. Go to sleep by 10 p.m.

This is a general schedule to ensure a balance of constructive activity and rest. Your daily schedule can be varied to include occasions for recreation and exercise, which should also be chosen to support your basic mind-body constitution. Regular routines are helpful for ordering your life and for creating and maintaining balance of biological functions.

Our approach is that we are spiritual beings in relationship to nature and nature's forces. Therefore, everything we do should result in more expanded awareness and improved function. Avoid becoming so fascinated by or preoccupied with procedures that you tend to forget your innate divinity and relationship with the Infinite.

Review, Memorize, and Comprehend
the Meanings of these Basic Words

One Sanskrit word can have a meaning that may require several words to describe. Learning these basic words and their meanings can be a consciousness-expanding experience, providing access to realms of knowledge beyond the reach of the mind. An easy way to become familiar with them is to read their definitions aloud.

- *Ayurveda* (i´-yur-vāde-a, or i´-yur-vāde) – Derived from *Ayur*, life; and *veda*, knowledge. *Veda* means "remembered" or "revealed" knowledge, with origins in Consciousness itself.
- *dosha* (doe´-sha) – A governing principle that influences and determines biological and psychological characteristics. When in balance, the three *doshas* support the body's tissues and functions. *Doshas* are

derived from element influences which are derived from the influences of the three attributes (*gunas*) of nature. The three *doshas* are *vata* (derived from ether and air elements), *pitta* (derived from fire and water elements), and *kapha* (derived from water and earth elements). When disturbed, or stronger or weaker in influence, their effects (also referred to as *doshas*) are manifested as obvious symptoms to be observed and corrected by appropriate, effective actions.

- *guna* (gu´-nah) – Attribute or quality of consciousness expressive in nature which regulates cosmic forces. *Sattva guna* is expansive and luminous; *rajas guna* is active and transformative; *tamas guna* is heavy and obscures *sattvic* and *rajasic* characteristics. These three primary qualities are present in the field of God and throughout nature as the universe.

Salutation to the Goddess of learning, through whose grace the knowledge of the universe reflected in the mirror of the intellect is realized by persons of virtuous acts.
– *Charaka Samhita* –

Basic Mind-Body Constitution Self-Evaluation Chart

Mark the dominant (1 only) description typical of you when you are rested and functioning well.

Characteristic	Vata (air)	Pitta (fire)	Kapha (water)
1. Body	( ) Narrow hips, shoulders	( ) Moderate	( ) Broad hips, shoulders
2. Body weight	( ) Thin, tendons show	( ) Medium	( ) Heavy
3. Endurance, strength	( ) Low, poor	( ) Fair	( ) High, good
4. Skin condition	( ) Dry, rough, cool, dark	( ) Soft, fair, oily, delicate, pink to red	( ) Oily, pale, moist, white
5. Skin, aging	( ) Dry, flaky, wrinkles	( ) Freckles, moles, pigmentation	( ) Smooth, few wrinkles
6. Hair	( ) Dry	( ) Medium	( ) Oily
7. Hair color	( ) Dark brown to black	( ) Light blond, red, light brown	( ) Medium blond, medium to dark brown
8. Hair texture	( ) Curly, kinky	( ) Wavy, fine, soft	( ) Strait or wavy, thick
9. Appetite, digestion	( ) Erratic, heavy, stays thin	( ) Sharp hunger	( ) Moderate, mild hunger
10. Teeth	( ) Large, protruding, crooked	( ) Yellowish, moderate	( ) White, large, little decay
11. Eyes	( ) Small, black or brown	( ) Hazel, green, grey	( ) Large, blue or brown
12. Bowel movements	( ) Dry, hard, constipation	( ) soft, oily, loose	( ) Heavy, slow, thick

13. Sex urge	( ) Frequent	( ) Moderate	( ) Cyclical, infrequent
14. Physical activity	( ) Flighty, restless	( ) Aggressive, focused	( ) Calm, steady
15. Voice, speech	( ) High pitched, fast, vibrato dissonant, weeping	( ) Medium-pitched, sharp, laughing	( ) Low-pitched, melodious, slow, monotone
16. Taste preferences	( ) Oily, heavy, sweet, soupy, salty, sour	( ) Medium, light, sweet, warm, bitter, astringent	( ) Dry, light, low-fat, sweet, pungent
17. Emotional state	( ) Insecure, unpredictable	( ) Aggressive, irritable	( ) Calm, agreeable
18. Sleep pattern	( ) Short, insomnia	( ) Sound, medium	( ) Deep, easy, prolonged
19. Memory	( ) Short-term	( ) Good, but not prolonged	( ) Long-term
20. Financial behavior	( ) Spends quickly and unwisely	( ) Saves, though impulsive	( ) Saves and accumulates
21. When threatened	( ) Fearful, anxious	( ) Angry, irritable, fights	( ) Indifferent, withdraws
22. Dreams while asleep	( ) Fear, flying, running	( ) Fire, strife, emotional	( ) Of water, erotic
23. Mental tendencies	( ) Questions, theorizes	( ) Judgmental, artistic	( ) Stable, logical
24. Quality of pulse	( ) Thready, slithering	( ) Moderate, jumping	( ) Slow and graceful
25. Pulse beats	( ) 80–100 times a minute	( ) 70–80 times a minute	( ) 60–70 times a minute
	Subtotal Vata times 4 = ____	**Subtotal Pitta** times 4 = ____	**Subtotal Kapha** times 4 = ____

The subtotals should add up to 100 percent. Write your basic mind-body constitutional type on page 25.

*Your Personal Application of
Life-Knowledge Program #1*

Apply what you know by examining your life. Choose a useful course of life-enhancing action and adhere to it. When you do this, knowledge is demonstrated and verified by your personal experiences. It becomes your own. Write clearly and thoughtfully your responses to the following questions and recommended procedures. Be honest and decisive. Follow through with alert participation. Be a dedicated doer.

1. Read this chapter again to acquire an intellectual grasp of the information. If a concept is not immediately understood, examine it until understanding is acquired. At a deep, soul level, you already know these life-knowledge principles.

2. Review, memorize, and comprehend the meanings of *Ayurveda*, *dosha*, *guna*, and any other words which are not familiar to you, until you are comfortable with them. It can be of help to write the words and their meanings and speak them. Speaking aloud will improve your powers of memory.

3. Be resolved to fulfill all of life's purposes. You can, if you sincerely want to. You have unlimited innate powers and abilities to awaken and actualize. The universe will support your aspirations and endeavors.

4. Refer to the chart on the previous pages to determine

your basic mind-body constitution. It is either *vata*, *pitta*, or *kapha*, *vata-pitta*, *vata-kapha*, *pitta-vata*, *pitta-kapha*, *kapha-vata*, *kapha-pitta*, or *vata-pitta-kapha*. Very seldom are the influences of the three *doshas* evenly balanced. List the dominant one first, followed by the others to determine the percentages of influences. _____

Remember your basic mind-body constitution as you read this book, being attentive to information that relates to it. Adopt the recommended practices and routines that can be helpful to you.

5. Write your needs, hopes, dreams, and aspirations. The first stage in the personal fulfillment process is to clearly define what you want to accomplish.

_____

_____

_____

_____

_____

_____

There are some people who respond with alert attention when you speak to them. That is the way of a true devotee. Thereafter, the devotee never looks back to the former sleep of delusion, but seeks ever greater wakefulness in God.
– *Paramahansa Yogananda* –

2

Guidelines to Understanding and Balancing the Mind-Body Constitution

While learning and applying various practical procedures for mind-body constitution balance, it is important to remember that our spiritual awareness is the primary, determining factor in the process. When spiritually awake, we are spontaneously inclined to live constructively and do what is most beneficial. Should a challenge then be present, we will quickly act to restore order and balance to every aspect of our lives.

Deficiency of spiritual awareness can result in intellectual errors, mental confusion, irrational thinking, moodiness, emotionalism, and an unnatural, disorganized lifestyle. Any or all of the psychological states and behaviors which are common when awareness is clouded and the mind is conditioned by delusions, illusions, obsessions, memories of pain or failure, and habits which are life-suppressing rather than life-enhancing, might be present. These can contribute to discomfort, weaken the body's immune system, and unsettle the actions of the three *doshas*: the primary governing influences that determine the states of the mind-body constitution.

The most effective approach to total wellness is a life-management program with thoughtful attention given to spiritual, psychological, and physical wellness, rather than concentrating on one aspect and paying little heed to the others. If we endeavor to cultivate spiritual awareness while psychological problems are ignored and everything else we do is not supportive of total wellness, results will usually be unsatisfactory. If we focus on physical routines while allowing our mental and emotional states to be disruptive or our spiritual practices to be sporadic or too passive, we will not experience the total benefits we desire and deserve. What is most supportive is a consciously chosen lifestyle which is wholesome, constructive, and results-oriented at all levels.

Three supportive matters to which to be attentive are food choices, sleep, and conservation and purposeful use of available energy. What we choose to eat, how we schedule our time so that sufficient rest is obtained to allow renewal, and whether or not we use our vital forces so they are not wasted but are used constructively, is revealing of our degree of self-esteem and of our commitment to healthy, meaningful living and spiritual growth.

To be healthy and functional, it is important that we have a clear sense of purpose for living and are resolved to that end. If we are not purposeful, if we do not know why we are living our lives, commitment to healthy living routines will be difficult. Mental conflicts and emotional confusion that contribute to disinterested or erratic behaviors in everyday circumstances will also interfere with our endeavors to help ourselves to actualize wholeness. Conscious selection of foods provides the opportunity to demonstrate our willingness to be self-responsible for our well-being. Thoughtless or careless actions in one aspect of our lives indicate a tendency toward indifference and other self-defeating attitudes which may also be characteristic of how we routinely behave.

Regular, sound sleep rests the mind and renews the body. Many of the body's circadian rhythms (Latin, *circa*, about: *dies*, day)—including the cycles of temperature, blood pressure, and hormone levels—can be disrupted because of irregular sleep patterns and lack of sleep. Some resulting life-suppressing effects may be tiredness, mental confusion, and impaired physical coordination. Sleep on a regular schedule in a dark, quiet place, awaken refreshed, and begin your day with alert, energetic, purposeful intention. You will be healthier and happier.

The Sanskrit word for conserving and constructively using vital forces is *brahmacharya* (*brahma*, divine; *charya*, going). The ideal is to direct all forces to life-enhancing purposes, including spiritual unfoldment. When vital forces are dissipated, mental powers are diminished, the body's immune system is weakened, and the *doshas* are unbalanced. Vital forces are dissipated by excesses of any kind: worry, anxiety, extreme effort to concentrate, restlessness, too much talking and laughing, overuse of any of the senses, ingestion of toxic substances, insufficient sleep or rest, too much socializing, and overwork. They are conserved by mental peace, emotional calmness, rational thinking, faith, moderate talking, prudent use of the senses, nourishing foods, sufficient sleep and rest, dispassion when interacting with others and the environment, relaxed accomplishment of purposes, meditation, and divine remembrance. Conserved vital forces are transmuted into subtle and fine essences to nourish the body and refine the brain and nervous system.

Some causes of discomfort or illness over which we have conscious control are: mental conflicts and psychological disturbances; excessive use of the senses and of the body; insufficient use of the senses and of the body; misuse of mental abilities, the senses, the body, and knowledge; and environmental factors.

We can learn by practice to be mentally calm, think rationally, and be emotionally settled. We can manage stress and avoid exhausting the physical systems. We can learn to wisely use our senses. We can choose a sensible wellness program to strengthen and enliven the body. We can choose to use the knowledge we have and acquire more by study, observation, and experience. We can choose wholesome, supportive environmental conditions and learn to adapt to seasonal changes.

Even conditions which may have a genetic basis or which were caused by accidents can be addressed and resolved. The important matter is to clearly understand that, as spiritual beings, we are in a position to implement intentional, causative influences which can change psychological, physical, and even environmental circumstances. *At the level of soul awareness there is nothing that needs to be healed. At this level we are ever serene and whole.* Established in soul awareness, we can do practical things to cause desirable adjustments in the outer realm. Acknowledge, speak, and soulfully realize:

> Because I am an individualized expression of divine consciousness, I am a life-giving spiritual being. My enlightened awareness energizes my mind, enlivens my body, and is the determining cause of harmonious, supportive, personal relationships and environmental conditions. Because I am always knowledgeably established in flawless understanding, I perceive accurately, think clearly, act wisely, and experience orderly unfoldments of events and circumstances

in all aspects of my life. The blessings I have
I thankfully and joyously wish for all people.
I am peaceful. I am happy.

It is important to cultivate spiritual awareness because
it impels thoughts and actions to be constructive, directly
and beneficially influences the mind and body, and
attracts supportive circumstances that nurture our lives.
Alert attention should also be directed to cultivating
healthy psychological states and attending to the needs
of the body. However, preoccupation with psychological
states and physical conditions that results in self-
centeredness is just as unwise as is neglect. Perceive your
mind for what it is: a creative medium with which to
interact with objective circumstances and with subjective
realities. Perceive your body for what it is: a vehicle
through which to express and experience life. Avoid thinking of yourself as a mind or as a body, for you are superior
to both. Preoccupation with the body can lead to obses-
sive behaviors, or to hypochondria (a persistent, neurotic
conviction that one is or is likely to become ill, often
involving perceptions and complaints of discomfort in the
absence of any supporting causes).

We are psychologically healthy when we are growing
steadily in the direction of emotional maturity. Every person born into the world must undergo progressive psychological transformations. When very young, we want
to discover who we are—to have an identity. As we grow
older, we attempt to be self-determined and to make our
way in the world by self-reliant endeavors. Eventually,
we aspire to understand our relationship with God. If our
intellectual and emotional unfoldment is slowed or

stopped, we become victims of arrested growth until learning and growing again proceed in the direction of full actualization of our mental and spiritual potential. A major obstacle to spiritual growth and to helping ourselves to overall wellness is a mental attitude which is resistant to change, supported by unwillingness to help ourselves once valid knowledge of how to do so has been acquired. It is helpful to understand that, except in extreme instances of disability, we are primarily responsible for our total wellness—for restoring ourselves to wellness if not yet completely well, and for remaining healthy and functional.

The Actions of the Three Doshas: the Primary, Governing Influences of Our Mind-Body Constitution

The primary governing influences of the mind-body constitution are expressive aspects of the five element influences, which are expressive aspects of the three constituents or attributes (*gunas*) of Consciousness which pervade the field of nature. Review the chart illustrating the categories of manifestation of Consciousness on page 12 until you have a clear understanding of the processes. Allow yourself time to fully understand the actions of the *gunas*, element influences, and governing influences or *doshas*. Knowledge of these aspects of life and their roles in regulating mental and physical states will unfold from within your own consciousness.

When we are fully enlightened, we can remove ourselves from the influences of the *doshas* and the *gunas*. Until then, so long as we are identified with individualized existence and a mind or physical body, we will have to cooperate with the influences which regulate nature's actions and processes.

Remember that *doshas* are subtle, influential forces. When their actions in our mind-body constitution are balanced, we experience psychological and physical wellness. When they are somewhat unbalanced, we may feel uneasy. When they are more obviously unbalanced—when one or more of the three *dosha* influences are excessive or deficient—discernible symptoms of unwellness can be observed and experienced.

Regardless of the percentages of *vata*, *pitta*, or *kapha* influences, your basic constitution represents your psychological and physical nature. When balance is maintained, health is optimum.

Some characteristics of the influences of the three *doshas* and ways restore and maintain balance are:

- *Vata Dosha*: *Vata* means "wind, to move, flow, direct the processes of, or command." It enables the other two *doshas* to be expressive. The actions of *vata* are drying, cooling, light, agitating, and moving. It sustains effort, inhalation and exhalation, circulation, movements of impulses, tissue balance, and coordination of the senses. Its primary seat or location in the body is the colon. It also resides in the hips, thighs, ears, and bones, and is related to touch sensation. *Vata*, being a combination of ether and air influences, is present and influential where there are spaces in which things (life force, thoughts, fluids, nerve impulses) can move.

  When vata dosha is disturbed or out of balance, some symptoms can be anxiety, worry, a tendency to overexertion, insomnia, chronic tiredness, mental and emotional depression, physical tension and other symptoms of stress, a weakened immune system, headaches, underweight, constipation, skin dryness, erratic flows of life force and nerve impulses, mental confusion, emotional conflict, inability to make decisions, impulsiveness, fast and disconnected speech, fantasy, illusions, and sensations of being lightheaded and removed from thoughts, feelings, or circumstances.

Indications of balanced vata influences are mental alertness and abundance of creative energy, good elimination of waste matters from the body, sound sleep, a strong immune system, enthusiasm, emotional balance, and orderly functioning of the body's systems.

People with a pronounced vata constitution or with a vata imbalance are advised to rest sufficiently, establish and maintain an orderly daily routine, and choose foods, behaviors, personal relationships, and environmental circumstances which can be instrumental in balancing *vata* characteristics. It is also important to regulate mental and physical impulses and to modify mental attitudes, emotional states, and behaviors in supportive ways.

Sweet, sour, and salty tastes decrease *vata* influences, so include these tastes if *vata* influences need to be diminished. Milk, wheat, rice, and some fruits and berries can provide sweet and sour tastes.

Regular exercise should be relaxed and moderate. Hatha yoga practice in a meditative mood is good, as are t'ai chi, walking, and swimming. Avoid strenuous, competitive, frantic activities.

When possible, associate with people who are

calmly purposeful. Practice simple *pranayama* to calm the mind and balance flows of life force in the body. Meditate every day for deep relaxation.

- *Pitta Dosha*: *Pitta* is "fire." It heats, digests, and is influential in chemical and metabolic transformations. It is related to our ability to "see"—to perceive with our eyes and to intellectually discern. Being a combination of fire and water element influences, it is present in the body in moisture and oils, and in the fluids of the digestive system and blood. *Pitta's* primary seat or location in the body is the small intestine. It also resides in the eyes, stomach, sebaceous glands, blood, lymph, and perspiration.

  When disturbed or out of balance, some symptoms might be excessive body heat, digestive problems, a tendency to be hostile or angry and controlling, impatience, a tendency to exert excessive effort to achieve goals, vision difficulties, and being prone to make errors in judgment because of mental confusion or because passion or emotion blurs powers of intellectual discernment.

  Indications of balanced pitta influences are strong powers of digestion, vitality, goal-setting inclinations, good problem-solving skills, keen powers of intelligence, decisiveness, boldness and courage, and a bright complexion.

  People with a pronounced pitta constitution or a pitta dosha imbalance are advised to live more moderately, cultivate purity of intentions and actions, and choose foods, attitudes, behaviors, personal relationships, and environmental circumstances which can be instrumental in balancing *pitta* characteristics.

Because sweet, bitter, and astringent tastes decrease *pitta* influences, include these in your food plan if *pitta* characteristics are too pronounced. Complex carbohydrates, milk, and some fruits are sweet; some green, leafy vegetables are bitter; beans and some green vegetables are astringent.

Do things that cool the mind, emotions, and body. Avoid conflicts. Cultivate the virtues of honesty, morality, kindness, generosity, and self-control.

- *Kapha Dosha*: A combination of water and earth influences, *kapha* is present in the body as moisture and dense substance. It holds things together. Mucus, for instance, indicates its influence. *Kapha dosha* provides nourishment, substance, and support, and makes up the mass of the body's tissues and its lubricating aspects. Its influence upon our psychological nature results in modesty, patience, ability to endure, courage, a tendency to forgive, mental calmness, and emotional stability.

  Kapha dosha effects are mostly cold, moist, heavy, and slow. In the blood and circulatory system, *kapha* influence is nourishing, *pitta* influence is energizing or heating, *vata* influence contributes to circulation. The balanced influences of the *doshas* result in good health and orderly functioning. The primary seat or location of *kapha dosha* in the body is the stomach. It also resides in lymph and fat. It is related to smell and taste sensation.

  When kapha dosha influences are disturbed or out of balance, symptoms might be nausea, lethargy, a feel-

ing of heaviness, chills, looseness of the limbs, cough-
ing, mucus discharges, breathing difficulties, and a
tendency to sleep too much. Other symptoms can be
inertia, congestion, stagnation, and circulation problems. There may be a tendency toward obesity. Bore-
dom, laziness, and mental dullness may be present.

Indications of balanced kapha influences are physical strength, a strong immune system, serenity, mental resolve, rational thinking, ability to conserve and
use personal resources, endurance, and adaptability.

*People with a pronounced kapha constitution or a
kapha dosha imbalance* are advised to be receptive to
useful change, renounce impediments to progress, be
intentional in implementing life-enhancing actions,
and choose foods, mental attitudes, behaviors, exercise routines, and relationships and environmental
circumstances which can be instrumental in balancing *kapha* characteristics.

Pungent, bitter, and astringent tastes decrease
kapha influences. Black pepper, ginger, cumin, chili,
and some other spices provide the pungent taste;
bitter is provided by some green leafy vegetables; and
some green vegetables and beans provide the astringent taste. Note that the taste that decreases a *dosha*
usually increases one or both of the other two. For
general purposes, mildly increase the proportion of
foods which are helpful while somewhat decreasing
the proportions of others—having a sampling of all
six tastes at your major meal.

Meditation can be more intensive for *kapha* constitutions than for *vata* or *pitta* constitutions. Schedule time every day for prayer and meditation.

The following quotation is from *Sushruta Samhita*:

> One whose *doshas* are in balance, whose appetite is good, whose tissues are functioning normally, whose excretions are in balance, and whose physiology, mind, and senses are always full of bliss [the joy of life-awareness], is called a healthy person.

Cooperating With Daily and Seasonal Rhythms

Because *dosha* influences are determined by the three *gunas* which regulate cosmic forces, their characteristics expressed in the environment can influence our mind-body constitution. We can be healthy and functional by cooperating with daily and seasonal rhythms. Daily phases during which *dosha* influences prevail are as follows:

- *Vata* is influential from 2 a.m. to 6 a.m. (or sunrise). Awaken before 6 a.m. to eliminate body wastes and be attuned to the lightness and free flowing energy of *vata dosha* influences.
- *Kapha* is influential from 6 a.m. (or sunrise) to 10 a.m. If possible, this is a suitable time to exercise because strength and stamina are at a peak level. It is also a good time to focus on work or activity that requires concentration and inner strength.
- *Pitta* is influential from 10 a.m. to 2 p.m. Because digestive fire is stronger during this phase, it is the ideal time to have your major meal of the day.
- *Vata* is influential from 2 p.m. to 6 p.m. (or sunset). Food and exercise should be light at this time of day.

- *Kapha* is influential from 6 p.m. (or after sunset) to 10 p.m. Retire for sleep before 10 p.m.
- *Pitta* is influential from 10 p.m. to 2 a.m.

Adapt to the seasonal changes in your region of the world by observing prevailing environmental conditions. Note these seasonal phases of *dosha* influences in the northern hemisphere:

- *Vata* influences are pronounced during the winter months from November to February when the weather is cold and dry. Especially during these months observe dietary and activity regimens which pacify or subdue mental and physical *vata* characteristics. Foods should be heavier and nourishing.

- *Kapha* influences are pronounced during the spring months from March to June when the weather is wet and moisture in nature replaces dryness. This is a good season of the year to implement a gentle body cleansing program and to observe dietary and activity regimens which pacify or subdue *kapha* characteristics. Foods that increase *pitta* influences can be chosen. This is also a good time to implement a more active exercise program. Be sure to stay warm and dry. Cultivate warm emotional states.

- *Pitta* influences are pronounced during the summer months from July to October when the weather is hot. Maintain dietary and activity regimens which subdue *pitta* characteristics. Foods should be light and wet.

You Can Help Yourself to Total Wellness and Functional Freedom

As a spiritual being, you need not be a helpless effect of causes external to your essential (spiritual) nature. Avoid thinking that your mental states, emotional states, physical condition, personal relationships, or routine circumstances are solely the result of causes over which you have no control. It is unwise to think or say that you are unable to choose how to experience your life. Even though imbalanced *dosha* influences can contribute to mental and emotional confusion and physical unrest, they can be regulated by improvement of spiritual awareness, conscious adjustments of mental and emotional states, and supportive lifestyle routines and behaviors. Whatever psychological or physiological characteristics you might presently be expressing, if they are not entirely life-enhancing, change them by choosing constructive behaviors.

Never affirm that you cannot help yourself to total wellness and functional freedom. At the core of your being, know that you are a free spirit. Nurture spiritual growth by reading authoritative philosophical literature— the writings of enlightened people rather than those of the unenlightened or misguided. Meditate regularly until your awareness is consciously established in superconscious tranquility, and learn to live with intentional purpose. Always be aware of the end results of your endeavors. Know why you do what you do. You will then more easily be self-motivated and goal-directed. You will be inspired to do whatever is necessary to be successful in your endeavors. When devoid of alert interest in life, without curiosity and drive, there may be a tendency to complacently drift, or to be uncaring and apathetic.

We were not born into this world to suffer, to continually cope with challenging conditions, or to struggle to survive. We are here to learn about ourselves and the universe, unfold our innate soul abilities and capacities, live successfully, and be agents of divine purposes. The sooner we acknowledge why we are here and do what we can to enable ourselves to fulfill our purposes, the healthier and happier we will be.

Life-knowledge, when clearly understood and intelligently applied, enables us to effectively fulfill all of our mundane purposes and our spiritual destiny. Our mundane purposes are related to the realm or field of nature. They are the duties and obligations we have to ourselves, others, and the environment. Our spiritual destiny is to awaken fully to Self-knowledge, God-realization, and liberation of consciousness. Mundane and transcendental purposes can be fulfilled simultaneously. Skillful living frees energies and resources to be used constructively. It is the very best spiritual practice because it includes everything we do and of which we are aware. Spiritual awareness expands our consciousness and removes us from delusions (the results of intellectual errors), illusions (misperceptions), and all other life-suppressing circumstances and influences.

A Guide to Daily Meditation Practice for Relaxation and Spiritual Growth

Everyone should daily sit to meditate. When you do this, avoid fantasy, emotionalism, strenuous effort, and mental passivity. For constructive results, remain alert, intentional, and attentive to the procedure.

Some benefits of regular meditation practice are:

- Stress symptoms are reduced.
- The immune system is strengthened.
- The nervous system is enlivened.
- Regenerative energies are awakened.
- Biologic aging processes are slowed.
- Thought processes are ordered, and organs, glands, and systems of the body are encouraged to function more harmoniously and efficiently.
- Spiritual growth is quickened.
- Appreciation for living is enhanced.

People who are not consciously interested in spiritual growth should daily practice meditation for the life-enhancing benefits. Spontaneous, progressive spiritual growth will then occur naturally.

1. *Sit in a Quiet Place* – In a comfortable chair, sit with spine and head erect to demonstrate clear intention and to remain alert. It is all right to sit on your bed or the floor with your legs crossed if you prefer this meditation posture and are comfortable.

2. *Pray in Your Own Way* – Imagine and feel that the Infinite Presence is within and around you (it is). Release any sense of independent selfhood. Contemplate wholeness. If you don't pray, at least open your mind and your being to the Infinite.

3. *Use a Meditation Technique* – Use any technique you know to be helpful. A simple procedure is to *mentally*

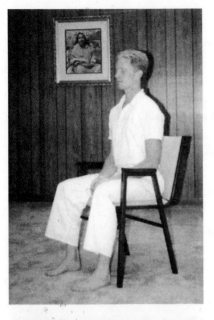

Established in a firm meditation posture, in a clean, appropriate place; there intent, with thoughts and senses controlled, one should practice meditation to purity the mind. With body, head, and neck erect, and motionless; gazing into the spiritual eye; serene, fearless, established in self-control, with mental impulses subdued, concentrating on the Supreme Reality, the devotee should sit, devoted to the highest realization.

The Bhagavad Gita
VI:11–14

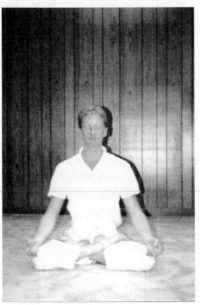

Photos: Two variations of postures suitable for the practice of meditation are illustrated here. Comfort should be assured for the purpose of undisturbed, alert contemplation.

"listen" to a pleasant word or word-phrase. When you breathe in, listen to the word or the first word of your word-phrase. When you breathe out, listen to the word or the second word of your word-phrase. A single word can be "peace," "light," or "God." A word-phrase can be "I am—peace," "I am—light," or "OM—God." Give your attention to the process, ignoring any shifting moods or thought processes. When you are relaxed and somewhat internalized, ignore the breathing cycle and listen to the inner, mental sound.

4. *Let Meditation Flow Spontaneously* – When mental peace is experienced, discard the practice of technique and rest in the tranquil silence. Your innate inclination to have awareness restored to wholeness will direct the meditation process. Surrender to it. Meditation will unfold spontaneously. Sit for at least twenty minutes for relaxation and absorption in superconscious peacefulness.

5. *Conclude the Session* – Meditate more than twenty minutes if you are inclined to do so. When you conclude your practice session, maintain awareness of yourself as a spiritual being as you attend to your chosen and necessary duties, routines, and relationships.

Once a week, twice a month, or once a month, on a regular schedule, meditate longer and deeper, resting in the aftereffects calm of meditation for as long as you feel inclined to do so. When you are physically relaxed and mentally and emotionally calm, superconsciousness will unfold. Superconsciousness is soul awareness, and is superior to ordinary states of wakefulness, sleep, or unconsciousness. Superconsciousness is redemptive. It purifies mind and body, unfolds innate understanding and spiritual qualities, and provides access to subjective knowledge of ourselves and of nature.

Remain Receptive and Responsive to Enlivening Flows of Consciousness

There is a benevolent Power nourishing our universe, and us, and we can learn to cooperate with it. To the extent that we are receptive and responsive to life, life is expressive through us as regenerative forces and around us as appropriate and supportive circumstances and events. Our spiritual forces flow freely when obstacles to their movements are absent. Do these things:

- Have the courage to live.
- Accept the fact that living can be spontaneous, fulfilling, and enjoyable.
- Be on friendly terms with a friendly universe and care for and nurture the planet.
- Make wise choices.
- Be appreciative of life's goodness and blessings.
- Demonstrate your compassion by serving others.
- Solve all problems with insightful understanding.
- Do everything you should do. Renounce behaviors that are not worthy of you.
- Don't pretend to be a victim of circumstances. You are a spiritual being endowed with limitless capacities for acquiring knowledge and skills.
- Educate yourself and be as knowledgeable and effec-

tively functional as you can be.

- Pray and meditate every day. Observe the teachings and practices of your religion or faith.
- Choose a lifestyle that is entirely supportive of you and your worthy purposes.
- Abide by the ways of righteousness: the spiritual, mental, and moral principles and laws of nature that provide a firm foundation for living.
- Wake up, grow up (be emotionally mature and responsible), perform your duties, fulfill your obligations, and flow in harmony with the rhythms of the universe.
- Be happy. Be thankful. Be soul-centered.

With attention focused on the object of contemplation, when the meditator becomes so identified with it that awareness of the personality-identity ceases, the state of perfect concentration [oneness] is accomplished.
    – *Swami Sri Yukteswar* –

Vata Dosha Characteristics
and Balancing Routines

When Balanced

Mental alertness, energetic, good powers of elimination, sound sleep, strong immune system, enthusiasm, imaginative, optimistic outlook on life, feelings of security and well-being.

When Disturbed

Anxiety, worry, tendency to overexertion, chronic fatigue, mental depression, emotional sadness, feelings of loneliness and insecurity, tension headaches, underweight, constipation, restless, scattered attention, fast and disconnected speech, erratic behaviors, unpredictable, questions things instead of learning and applying what is learned for practical results.

To Restore and Maintain Balance

It is important to obtain adequate rest and maintain regular lifestyle routines. Begin with positive intention and definite resolve, then follow through with confidence. Appropriate, constructive actions will produce satisfying results.

Cultivate mental calm, emotional peace, and optimism. To neutralize a tendency to be "spaced-out," do things that are centering and grounding. Avoid attitudes, feelings, behaviors, and relationships which increase *vata* characteristics.

Sweet, sour, and salty tastes decrease *vata* influences. Milk, rice, wheat, and some berries and fruits are sweet and have a sweet post-digestive taste.

Regular exercise should be relaxed and moderate. Hatha yoga in a meditative mood is good; also t'ai chi, walking, and swimming. Avoid activities which are too strenuous.

When possible, associate with people who are calmly purposeful. Learn and practice simple *pranayama* to calm the mind and balance the flows of life force in the body.

Meditate in a relaxed, surrendered manner every day.

Pitta Dosha Characteristics
and Balancing Routines

When Balanced

Strong powers of digestion, energetic, keen intellect, bright complexion, goal-oriented, decisive, successful in endeavors.

When Disturbed

Excessive body heat, hostile, controlling, quick to anger, impatient, overly aggressive, problems with vision and perhaps with "seeing" solutions to problems, restlessness, unsettled sleep pattern. May tend to be addicted to substances or behaviors as a way of blocking out frustration or a sense of failure.

How to Restore and Maintain Balance

As recommended for all three mind-body constitutions, attention should be given to life management routines. To have a clear knowledge of purpose, be sure you know why you do what you do. Be aware that you are living your life in relationship with the Infinite. Cultivate an attitude of being a useful agent for constructive accomplishment. Avoid ego-fixation.

Cultivate serenity and emotional calm. Avoid mental attitudes, feelings, behaviors, and relationships which stimulate and increase *pitta* (hot, fiery) characteristics.

Sweet, bitter, and astringent tastes decrease *pitta* influences; include these in your food plan. Complex carbohydrates, milk, and some fruits are sweet; some green leafy vegetables are bitter; beans and some green vegetables are astringent.

Exercise should be relaxed and moderate. Hatha yoga, t'ai chi, walking, swimming, bicycling, tennis, golf, and any other enjoyable activity can be helpful. Exercise for enjoyment and a sense of well-being. Avoid being overly competitive.

Do things which cool the mind, emotions, and body. Avoid conflicts. Attend to meaningful regimens. Cultivate the virtues of honesty, morality, kindness, generosity, self-control, continued learning, and insightful living, understanding that you are cooperating with a Larger Purpose. Meditate daily.

Kapha Dosha Characteristics and Balancing Routines

When Balanced

Calm, rational, good powers of endurance, prudent manager of personal responsibilities and resources, compassionate, long-range views, strong immune system, and dependable.

When Disturbed

A tendency to be overweight and lethargic, slow digestion, physical discomfort may be related to body structure and joints, excess mucus, and other water-earth characteristics. Psychological characteristics may include greediness and attachment, in contrast to the more balanced characteristics of acquiring and responsibly managing material resources for necessary, worthwhile, and benevolent purposes.

How to Restore and Maintain Balance

Inertia, if present, should be neutralized by choosing to implement constructive actions. Move ahead by renouncing everything that restrains or confines. Become more expansive in mental outlook. Motivate yourself when necessary.

Cultivate awareness of your relationship with life as wholeness. Adopt psychological characteristics and behaviors opposite of those which are characteristic of imbalanced *kapha dosha* influences. Do not resist the idea of useful change.

Pungent, bitter, and astringent tastes decrease *kapha* influences. Black pepper, ginger, cumin, chili, and some other spices provide the pungent taste, bitter is provided by some green leafy vegetables, and some green vegetables and beans provide the astringent taste. *Note that the tastes which decrease a dosha, increase one or both of the other two.* For general purposes, mildly increase the proportion of foods which are helpful while decreasing the others—having a sampling of all six tastes at each major meal.

Regular exercise can be a little more intensive than for *vata* or *pitta* constitutions. Pray and meditate every day.

Your Personal Application of
Life-Knowledge Program #2

1. Write a general lifestyle routine designed to assist you
    to maintain your basic mind-body constitution balance.

_____

_____

_____

2. Write your daily meditation schedule: time, duration,
    and practice routine. Practice regularly, without anxi-
    ety about results. Benefits will naturally unfold.

_____

_____

3. Write a list of constructive behaviors or circumstances
    to which you want to give more attention: mental
    attitude, emotional stability, good health habits, work
    or activity habits, relationships, and whatever else
    seems to you to be necessary or worthwhile.

_____

_____

_____

_____

4. Write a list of self-defeating or life-inhibiting behaviors or circumstances you choose to overcome by renouncing or replacing them with entirely constructive behaviors and circumstances. Do everything you can to be receptive and responsive to enlivening flows of consciousness and supportive circumstances.

_____

_____

_____

5. Be still for a few moments, then write a clearly worded affirmation that accurately defines your decision to live wholesomely and constructively. As you do this, remember that you are a spiritual being with free choice and unlimited potential to unfold and experience your highest good in all aspects of life.

_____

_____

_____

The origin of the vital force which courses through the body is self-begotten, and is regarded as identical with the divine energy of the Eternal Life (God) because it is unconditioned and absolute in its actions and effects.
– *Sushruta Samhita* –

3

Choosing Foods and Behaviors for Inner Balance and Spiritual Growth

The governing principles which regulate biological processes and influence psychological states pervade the universe because Consciousness, the basis of the natural order, is omnipresent. We are wise to learn about them because their influences are expressive in our minds and bodies, the foods we eat, and the environment.

Learning and growing require that we be willing to adjust our way of looking at circumstances, accept new ideas when they are perceived as valid, apply helpful principles and procedures to nurture total well-being, and live as skillfully and as effectively as possible.

Transformational experiences require that we be willing, when necessary, to undergo rapid improvement even if radical changes are necessary. Instead of thinking about what might have to be given up in order to awaken to a higher level of understanding or to demonstrate improved functional skills and be restored to wholeness, a more constructive attitude is to visualize the desirable outcomes of our wisely chosen actions.

When knowledgeably engaged in intentional actions, it is helpful to carry in our awareness a mental picture of end results. Doing this will facilitate expansion of awareness, awaken dormant soul forces, stimulate flows of inspiration and streams of creative ideas, release energy for constructive use, and provide motivation to focus on matters essential to accomplish chosen purposes.

While engaged in intentional actions, at the deepest level of your being know the idealized outcome to be a certainty. Then, whatever you do will allow desired results to be demonstrated. You will be decisive, insightful, and successful. Favorable circumstances and cooperative forces of nature will be attracted into your life to assist and support your endeavors.

Whenever you need to renounce a mental attitude, belief, opinion, mood, habit, behavior, relationship, or action, know that you are but sacrificing the lesser for the greater, the lower for the higher. With understanding, it will be easier to make constructive, life-enhancing choices and abide by them. With each overcoming, the spiritual power that was suppressed by former, unwholesome habits and behaviors, will be released for constructive purposes. Day by day, week by week, year by year, your understanding will increase. Your ability to live effectively will rapidly improve. Grace will bless your life beyond the limits of the mind to imagine.

The Five Subtle Aspects of Vata (air) Dosha

For general purposes, to balance the *doshas* it is not necessary to know the five subtle aspects of each of them, but it can be helpful to have this knowledge when specific conditions need to be addressed. This knowledge also improves our understanding of nature's processes.

The soul's life force (*prana*) blends with the physical body at the base of the brain, at the medulla oblongata. From there, it flows to the higher brain and down into the body through the vital centers (*chakras*) along the spinal pathway. From the *chakras*, life force is distributed through channels (*nadis*) to enliven the physiology. Although life force is nonphysical, it relates to and acts upon organic matter. As life force becomes involved with the body, it expresses as different frequencies to perform various functions:

- *Prana, the Primary Aspect*: Seated in the brain. It governs swallowing and inhalation. It regulates operations of the senses, mental processes, the heart, and our states of consciousness. It enables us to draw in universal life force through the medulla oblongata. The other four aspects of *prana* are derived from this primary aspect. (*Pra*, forth; *an*, to breathe.)
- *Upward Moving (udana) Aspect*: Seated in the throat and active in the chest. It governs speech and exhalation. It contributes to lifting vital forces toward the higher brain when meditating, to expansion of consciousness when we aspire to transcendent realizations, and to the soul's withdrawal from the body at the time of transition. During meditation, when the body is relaxed and mental processes and life forces are calmed and balanced, breathing becomes slow, smooth and refined, and awareness becomes clear. This occurs naturally when our attention is effortlessly absorbed in contemplation. It can be facilitated by the practice of *pranayama* before meditation. (*Ud*, up; *a*, toward; *an*, to breathe.)
- *Equalizing (samana) Aspect*: Seated in the small intestine. It governs digestion, assimilation, and biochemical processes. (*Sama*, equal; *an*, to breathe.)

- *Pervasive (vyana) Aspect*: Seated in the heart region and flowing throughout the body. It governs the circulatory system and movements of muscles and joints, discharges internal secretions, resists decay, and maintains balance. (*Vi*, apart; *a*, towards; *an*, to breathe.)
- *Downward Moving (apana) Aspect*: Centered in the colon. It governs elimination of the body's waste products, menstruation, childbirth, and expulsion of reproductive fluids. (*Apa*, away; *an*, to breathe.)

Mental confusion, emotional unrest, erratic lifestyle routines, overexertion, and any kind of trauma including accidents which cause injury, fright, or pain, can imbalance flows of life force in the body. Mental calmness and orderly thinking, emotional balance, regulated lifestyle routines, stress management, optimism, meditation, and relaxed, purposeful living help to maintain balanced flows of the body's life forces.

The Five Subtle Aspects of Pitta (fire) Dosha

- *The Fire of Digestion*: Seated in the small intestine. It is the primary *pitta* aspect from which the other four are derived. Efficient powers of digestion are necessary to begin the body's food transformation processes. Digestive fire can be enlivened by the use of specific herbs, by general improvement of health, and by *pranayama* routines and hatha yoga practices which act directly upon the lumbar *chakra* and solar plexus.
- *The Knowledge Fire*: Seated in the brain and heart region. It is related to powers of intellectual discernment and our ability to efficiently plan and accom-

plish goals and fulfill purposes.

- *The Radiance Fire*: Seated in the skin. It influences complexion and governs the processing of heat.
- *The Fire of Visual Perception*: Seated in the eyes. It governs the reception of light and ability to see.
- *The Fire of Coloring*: Seated in the liver. Influential in the blood, stomach, spleen, and small intestine. It governs the coloring of bile, blood, and body wastes.

The author of *Charaka Samhita* describes the actions of fire (*agni*) in the body as governing general appearance, strength, energy, health, and increase of body weight.

Pitta dosha is the energy of fire; *agni* is the manifestation of the biological fire. Excess *kapha dosha* slows digestive processes. When *pitta dosha* is influential, digestive powers are strong. When *vata dosha* interferes with the biological fire, digestive powers are irregular.

The Five Aspects of Kapha (water-earth) Dosha

- *The Aspect of Calming*: Seated in the brain, manifested as cerebrospinal fluid, and in the heart region as subtle essence. Its influence contributes to mental calmness and emotional stability, and it is related to memory.
- *The Aspect of Lubrication*: Manifested as synovial fluid in the joints of the bones.
- *The Aspect of Moistening*: Manifested as secretions of the mucus lining of the stomach and elsewhere. In the stomach it contributes to liquefying food during preliminary stages of digestion.
- *The Perception Aspect*: Seated in the mouth and tongue, and manifested as saliva that assists tasting

of foods. Saliva and taste sensation make important contributions to preliminary stages of digestion. Saliva mixed with food begins the process of digestion. The taste of food is directly transmitted to the brain, which signals the body to respond.

* *The Aspect of Support*: Seated in the lungs and heart region. The basis of phlegm and the other actions of *kapha dosha* in the body, and corresponds to the primary watery essence (plasma) distributed by the actions of the heart and lungs.

There are several kinds of interactions of influences that can affect our circumstances: (1) the *doshas* are the primary influential principles that affect the mind as well as the body and can be regulated by employing specific actions and routines; (2) our psychological states can directly influence our physical states by the kind and quality of our thoughts, by the kind and quality of our emotions, and by our actions and reactions determined by our psychological states; (3) physical states can influence our mental and emotional states and, if we allow them to do so, our states of spiritual awareness. When the *doshas* are imbalanced, we may demonstrate corresponding symptoms of discomfort or confusion. To maintain stability a positive approach to life management and intentional living should be established in Self-knowledge (soul awareness). All practical actions to facilitate wellness and efficient functioning of mind and body should be implemented. Harmonious relationships with people, creatures, and the environment should be cultivated.

The Supporting Tissues of the Body and Our Interactions with the Universe

We are spiritual beings relating to nature through mind and body. Our essential being is nonmaterial. The mind is formed of subtle matter and the body is formed of gross matter. When the mind is devoid of conflicts and is no longer disturbed by external influences, *sattva guna* (the attribute of clarity and illumination) is the ruling influence of its actions. The influences of clarity and illumination should extend to the body so that total wellness is naturally and spontaneously experienced.

The currents of life are inclined to flow. When their flows are impeded or blocked, *tamas guna* becomes the more influential attribute. Stagnation and inertia become the determining factors until *sattvic* influences supported by the actions of *rajas guna* overcome heaviness, as light removes darkness. We participate with the processes of Spirit and nature. Spirit, the enlivening life of God, is ever inclined to transform nature and awaken souls. The universe is the result of interactions between God as Spirit and God's creative energies as nature. Everything in manifestation is included in God's field of Consciousness. Nature is God's creative energy expressing.

Our minds are portions (particularized units) of Cosmic or Universal Mind. The ingredients of nature comprise our bodies. We have outlived several bodies during our current sojourn on earth because the atoms and cells of the body are constantly being replaced. The atoms of our bodies were formed in the stars eons ago. Our bodies are energy forms vitalized by life force and nourished by foods we eat.

When we are self-conscious (egocentric), we may erroneously believe ourselves to be a habit-bound personality or a mere mass of flesh. We may mistakenly presume ourselves to be at the mercy of our conditioned mental processes, arrested emotional states, physical conditions, or personal circumstances. When we are strongly identified with these opinions, we are deluded (have incorrect beliefs about ourselves and life processes) as a result of intellectual errors—which can be corrected. By acquiring accurate information, and testing it by personal application, we can banish delusions and remove ourselves from their effects.

Ayurvedic literature describes seven tissues (*dhatus*) of the body as products of food transformation:

- *Plasma (rasa)*: Carries nutrients of digested food to nourish tissues, organs, and systems of the body.
- *Blood (rakta)*: Carries oxygen and nutrients to the tissues and waste products away from them. Blood, poured into a test tube and treated with salt, separates into three distinct layers. At the top is plasma, a clear, golden liquid. In the middle is a solid band of white cells. At the bottom is a thick band of red cells.
- *Muscle (mamsa)*: Covers vital organs, moves joints, helps in maintaining bodily strength, plays a role in metabolic processes.
- *Fat (meda)*: Lubricates the tissues.
- *Bone (asthi)*: Supports body structures.
- *Marrow (maja)*: In the bone hollows. Produces blood cells and platelets which repair blood vessels.
- *Reproductive Tissue (shukra)*: The final physical manifestation of food transformation.

The eighth manifestation of food transformation is a fine essence (*ojas*) at the juncture between consciousness and matter which is enlivening and regenerative. Its influence strengthens the body's immune system and imparts the radiance of vital health. It energizes the mind, contributes to powers of concentration and intellectual discernment, manifests as spiritual magnetism, and empowers resolve to experience rapid spiritual unfoldment and liberation of consciousness.

The Effects of Tastes and Subtle Properties of Foods

The six tastes of food are derived from the five element influences: ether, air, fire, water, and earth (refer to the chart in chapter 1 which shows the relationships of element influences to taste characteristics). The tastes derived from the specific element influences will increase those influences in the mind and body; the other tastes will decrease them. To strengthen the *doshas*, choose foods with the tastes which influence them. To reduce *dosha* effects, choose the other tastes:

- *Sweet*: Derived from water and earth element influences. It increases *kapha dosha* and reduces *vata* and *pitta*. Examples of foods with sweet taste are grains and other complex carbohydrates, milk, butter, and concentrated sugars. Sweet taste is best obtained from complex carbohydrates and complex sweeteners (in moderation) so that their post-digestive effects are the result of digestion. Concentrated sugars shock the body. When sweet taste is in the mouth, the brain immediately signals for a release of insulin into the blood stream to regulate sugar before food is digested. Concentrated sweet taste is not recommended (especially not refined sugar or sugar substitutes found in many soft drinks and other commercially prepared foods). The sweet taste of ordinary foods nourishes and builds the body. Many of the foods recommended for rejuvenation purposes are sweet when well-masticated and have a sweet post-digestive effect.

- *Sour*: Derived from fire and earth elements. It increases *pitta* and *kapha* and decreases *vata*. Some foods with sour taste are citrus and some other fruits, hard cheeses, and yogurt. Needed in small quantities.

- *Salty*: Derived from fire and water element influences. It increases *pitta* and *kapha* and decreases *vata*. Helps in maintaining mineral balance and retaining water. Can usually be derived from foods.

- *Pungent*: Derived from air and fire element influences. Increases *vata* and *pitta* and reduces *kapha*. Is in hot peppers, ginger, cumin, and some other spices. Needed for metabolism, stimulates appetite and digestion.

- *Bitter*: Derived from ether and air element influences. It increases *vata* and decreases *pitta* and *kapha*. Found in spinach and some other green leafy vegetables, eggplant, and turmeric. Helpful in detoxification of the body, hence its use in some medicinal preparations when body cleansing is needed.

- *Astringent*: Derived from ether and earth element influences. It increases *vata* and decreases *pitta* and *kapha*. Found in beans, lentils, and some fruits. Helpful in maintaining tissue firmness.

Foods also provide the following subtle qualities:

- *Heavy*: Increases *kapha*, decreases *vata* and *pitta*. Some sources are cheese, yogurt, and wheat products.
- *Light*: Increases *vata* and *pitta*, decreases *kapha*. Some sources are barley, apples, spinach, and corn.
- *Oily*: Increases *kapha*, decreases *vata* and *pitta*. Some sources are fatty foods, oils, and most dairy products.
- *Dry*: Increases *vata* and *pitta*, decreases *kapha*. Some sources are barley, corn, beans, and potatoes.
- *Hot*: Increases *pitta*, decreases *vata* and *kapha*. Obtained from hot foods and drinks.
- *Cold*: Increases *vata* and *kapha*, decreases *pitta*. Obtained from cold foods and drinks.

How different foods affect us depends upon their varied characteristics. When we are in good health, our knowledge of how foods may influence us and our instinctual inclinations can enable us to choose the best food plan. It can be helpful to be familiar with the following information. (*Note*: PDE means post-digestive effect.)

Apple: Sweet, astringent. Cooling. Sweet PDE. Light, rough. Increases *vata*, decreases *pitta*. All right for *kapha* constitution in moderate quantities.
Banana: Sweet, astringent. Cooling. Sour PDE. Smooth, heavy, laxative when taken in quantity. Increases *pitta* and *kapha*, decreases *vata*.
Coconut: Sweet. Cooling. Sweet PDE. Oily, smooth. Increases *kapha*, decreases *vata* and *pitta*.
Date (ripe): Sweet. Cooling. Sweet PDE. Oily. Decreases *pitta*. Dates, almonds, and honey with milk that has been boiled and cooled to a warm temperature is strengthening and

rejuvenating. To one cup of milk, add two ripe, pitted dates, a dozen almonds that have soaked in water overnight to soften (or one tablespoon of fresh almond butter), and a teaspoon of honey. Blend and drink slowly.

Fig: Sweet, astringent. Cooling. Sweet PDE. Heavy, nourishing. Increases *kapha*, decreases *vata* and *pitta*.

Grapes (purple): Sweet, sour, astringent. Cooling. Sweet PDE. Smooth, watery. Increases *kapha*, decreases *vata* and *pitta*.

Melon: Sweet. Cooling. Sweet PDE. Heavy, watery. Decreases *vata* and *pitta*.

Orange: Sweet, astringent. Heating. Sweet PDE. Heavy, promotes appetite. Increases *pitta* and *kapha*, decreases *vata*.

Peach: Sweet, astringent. Heating. Sweet PDE. Heavy, watery. Increases *pitta* and *kapha*, decreases *vata*.

Pear: Sweet and astringent. Cooling. Sweet PDE. Heavy, dry, rough. Increases *vata*, decreases *pitta* and *kapha*.

Plum: Sweet, astringent. Heating. Sweet PDE. Heavy, watery. Increases *pitta* and *kapha*, decreases *vata*.

Beet: Sweet. Heating. Sweet PDE. Heavy, smooth. In excess can increase *pitta* and *kapha*. Decreases *vata*.

Broccoli: Sweet, astringent. Cooling. Pungent PDE. Rough, dry. Increases *vata*, decreases *pitta* and *kapha*.

Cabbage: Sweet, astringent. Cooling. Pungent PDE. Rough, dry. Increases *vata*, decreases *pitta* and *kapha*.

Carrot: Sweet, bitter, astringent. Cooling. Pungent PDE. Heavy. In excess increases *pitta*. Decreases *vata* and *kapha*.

Cauliflower: Astringent. Cooling. Pungent PDE. Rough, dry. Increases *vata*, decreases *pitta* and *kapha*.

Celery: Astringent. Cooling. Pungent PDE. Rough, dry, light. Increases *vata*, decreases *pitta* and *kapha*.

Garlic: Pungent. Heating. Pungent PDE. Oily, smooth, heavy. Increases *pitta*, decreases *vata* and *kapha*.

Ginger: Pungent. Heating. Sweet PDE. Light, dry, rough. In excess it increases *pitta*. Decreases *vata* and *kapha*.

Lettuce: Astringent. Cooling. Pungent PDE. Cooling. Light. Increases *vata*, decreases *pitta* and *kapha*.

Raw onion: Pungent. Heating. Pungent PDE. Heavy, stimulating, strengthening. Increases *vata* and *pitta,* reduces *kapha.*

Potato: Sweet, salty, astringent. Cooling. Sweet PDE. Rough, dry, light. Increases *vata*, decreases *pitta* and *kapha.*

Spinach: Astringent. Cooling. Pungent PDE. Rough, dry. Increases *vata* and *pitta*, decreases *kapha.*

Sprouts: Mildly astringent. Cooling. Sweet PDE. Light. Suitable for all constitutions. In excess, may aggravate *vata.*

Tomato: Sweet, sour. Heating. Sour PDE. Light, moist. Increases all three *doshas.*

Zucchini Squash: Sweet, astringent. Cooling. Sweet PDE. Wet, light. May increase *kapha*, decreases *pitta*, all right for *vata.*

Barley: Sweet, astringent. Cooling. Sweet PDE. Light. Increases *vata*, decreases *pitta* and *kapha.*

Basmati Rice: Sweet. Cooling. Sweet PDE. Light, soft, smooth, nourishing. Decreases *vata* and *pitta*. All right for *kapha* constitution in moderation.

Brown Rice: Sweet. Heating. Sweet PDE. Heavy. Increases *pitta* and *kapha*, decreases *vata.*

Buckwheat: Sweet, astringent. Heating. Sweet PDE. Light, dry. Increases *vata* and *pitta*, decreases *kapha.*

Corn: Sweet. Heating. Sweet PDE. Light, dry. Increases *vata* and *pitta*, decreases *kapha.*

Oats: Sweet. Heating. Sweet PDE. Heavy. Dry oats increase *vata* and *pitta*, decrease *kapha*. Cooked oats increase *kapha*, decrease *vata* and *pitta.*

Millet: Sweet. Heating. Sweet PDE. Light, dry. Increases *vata* and *pitta*, decreases *kapha.*

Rye: Sweet, astringent. Heating. Sweet PDE. Light, dry. Increases *vata* and *pitta*, decreases *kapha.*

Wheat: Sweet. Cooling. Sweet PDE. Heavy. Increases *kapha*, decreases *vata* and *pitta.*

Almonds: Sweet. Heating. Sweet PDE. Heavy, oily. Increases *pitta* and *kapha*, decreases *vata.*

Cashews: Sweet. Heating. Sweet PDE. Heavy, oily. Increases *pitta* and *kapha*, decreases *vata.*

Peanuts: Sweet, astringent. Heating. Sweet PDE. Heavy, oily. Increases *pitta* and *kapha*. All right for *vata* in moderation. Difficult to digest. Should not be given to children before age six, and only in moderation after that.

Pumpkin Seed: Sweet, bitter, astringent. Heating. Pungent PDE. Heavy, dry. Increases *pitta* and *kapha*, decreases *vata*.

Sunflower Seed: Sweet, astringent. Heating. Sweet PDE. Heavy, oily. Mildly increases *pitta* and *kapha*, decreases *vata*.

Lentils: Sweet, astringent. Cooling. Sweet PDE. Dry, rough, heavy. Increases *vata* and *kapha*, decreases *pitta*.

Mung Beans: Sweet, astringent. Cooling. Sweet PDE. Light, soft. Increases *kapha*, reduces *vata* and *pitta*.

Soy Beans: Sweet, astringent. Cooling. Sweet PDE. Heavy, oily, smooth. Increases *vata* and *kapha*, decreases *pitta*.

Honey: Sweet, astringent. Heating. Sweet PDE. Dry, rough, heavy. Mildly increases *pitta*, decreases *vata* and *kapha*.

Sesame Oil: Sweet, bitter, astringent. Heating. Sweet PDE. Heavy, oily, smooth. Increases *pitta*, decreases *vata*. All right for *kapha* constitution in moderation.

Sunflower Oil: Sweet. Cooling. Sweet PDE. Light, oily, strengthening. All right for all three *doshas*.

Safflower Oil: Sweet, pungent. Heating. Pungent PDE. Light, sharp, oily, irritating if used excessively. Increases *pitta*, decreases *vata* and *kapha*.

Corn Oil: Sweet. Heating. Sweet PDE. Light, oily, smooth. Increases *pitta*. All right in moderation for *vata* and *kapha*.

Ghee (Clarified Butter): Sweet. Cooling. Sweet PDE. Light, oily, smooth. In moderation, useful for all *doshas*. Excessive use increases *kapha*. It promotes digestion, is strengthening, and is useful in transporting herbal influences to tissues.

Goat Milk: Sweet, astringent. Cooling. Sweet PDE. Light. Increases *vata*, decreases *pitta* and *kapha*. Usually more easily digested than cow milk for people who have difficulty with it.

Cow milk: Sweet. Cooling. Sweet PDE. Light, oily, smooth. Increases *kapha*, decreases *vata* and *pitta*. Milk is more easily digested if boiled and allowed to cool to a warm temperature before drinking.

With repeated study of these principles and experimentation with them, an understanding of the effects of tastes and the qualities of foods will be acquired. To maintain *dosha* balance, choose foods which are most suitable for your basic mind-body constitution, remembering to have the six tastes represented at each major meal while reducing the portions of foods which might cause imbalance. Except in extreme instances of imbalance, any of the foods listed in the charts at the end of this chapter may be consumed regardless of your basic constitution, with smaller portions of the ones which are not recommended for your basic constitution. Avoid fanaticism. When you are relaxed and healthy, your sense of what is best for you can be followed. When your body needs certain tastes and food quality influences, you may crave foods which can supply them. Learn to discriminate between cravings impelled by real needs and those which may have only a psychological basis.

Food should be fresh and clean, devoid of pesticide residues and in the most available natural state before preparation. It is a good idea to avoid overly processed foods, and foods with additives of all kinds, especially preservatives. If some foods are not compatible with your system, avoid them. Prepare meals with alert awareness of what you are doing, and why.

Eat in a relaxed manner, thankful for nature's gift of food and for the knowledge you have of your relationship with God and the universe. It is best to prepare food only for the meal for which it is intended and not save it for future use, except for foods which may satisfactorily be refrigerated for a day or two. Fresh foods are *sattvic*: they are nourishing and life-enhancing. Stale foods are *tamasic* because the life force is diminished or absent.

Consume only the quantity of food needed; it will be more efficiently processed by the body, conserving energy and resulting in feelings of lightness and well-being. When eating is a conscious, appropriate activity, there is less likelihood of excessive waste matters being produced. Foods which are not completely digested and transformed leave residues which must be eliminated. If waste matters remain in the body they can disrupt normal biological functions and cause discomfort and illness. The Ayurvedic term for the accumulation of excessive waste matters is *ama*, said to be sticky, white, and sometimes injurious to the body. When its presence is known, it should be eliminated.

The body's organs for elimination of waste matters are the colon, urinary tract, skin (through which perspiration, some oily substances, and other exudations are eliminated), and lungs (removal of carbon dioxide and other gaseous substances from blood). Have regular bowel movements. Eliminate urine when the urge to do so is present. Keep the skin clean by regular skin brushing and bathing. Learn to breathe correctly.

Elimination of toxic mental attitudes and emotional states which poison the mind, interfere with normal biological functions, and disturb *dosha* balance is as important as elimination of physical waste matters. Pessimism and fear are cold and increase *vata* characteristics. Frustration and anger are hot, sour, and bitter and increase *pitta* characteristics. Disinterest and apathy are heavy and increase *kapha* characteristics. Jealousy, envy, guilt, self-righteousness, deviousness, and all other mental and emotional disturbances are destructive and life-suppressing. Love, humility, compassion, and the tranquility of meditation are sweet and nourishing.

We should intentionally cultivate only constructive and life-enhancing mental and emotional states and qualities. We can do this by decisive choice and by implementing wholesome lifestyle regimens which support the choices we make. Mental and emotional states are more easily regulated when constructive actions are synchronized with thoughts and feelings.

As we awaken from self-consciousness and a false sense that life is fragmented, to clear awareness of wholeness, we experience episodes of growth and discovery which remind us that, this side of the Field of Pure Existence-Being, our possibilities for growth and Self-discovery are almost endless.

The Harmful Effects of Free Radicals and the Possible Usefulness of Vitamin Supplementation

An oxygen atom missing an electron (a free radical) attracts one from another atom. The atom from which an electron has been taken then needs to acquire one from another atom. The chain reaction results in cell damage, immune deficiency, and impaired biological function. Some vitamins have been found to be effective in partially controlling free radical damage, especially vitamins C and E. They are most efficiently utilized by the body when acquired from fresh foods. Have a variety of colorful vegetables and fruits in your daily diet. Choose supplements from natural sources: at least 500 milligrams of Vitamin C and 300 units of Vitamin E. Vitamin A, while useful as an antioxidant, is best obtained from foods which have other nutrients which enable the body to process it more effectively. Some recent research indicates that Vitamin A in supplement form is not as helpful as it was once thought it might be. Excessive use of Vitamin A supplements should be avoided by pregnant women. Research done in early 1996 indicated a possible link between daily intake of more than 5,000 International Units and some kinds of birth defects.

Vitamin supplements (and herbs), if used, should be thoughtfully and knowledgeably chosen. Near the end of the 20th century a published estimate of the amount of money spent annually in the United States on vitamins, minerals, and herbal products was approximately six billion dollars. Many people who use these products unwisely or excessively, are doing themselves more harm than good. Always be wary of hyperbole (extravagant claims), faddish trends, aggressive marketing programs, and unusually high prices.

A person's faith (that which one respects or defers to)
is in accord with the basic nature. One's personality and
circumstances are the result of preferred attitudes and
actions of the past; present states and conditions are the
result of what is presently believed and done.
– *The Bhagavad Gita (VII:3)* –

A Food Plan to Balance Vata Dosha

These guidelines can be used for *vata* mind-body constitutions, to maintain *dosha* balance, and to restore balance if necessary, regardless of the basic constitution. *Vata* influences the movement of thoughts, feelings, *prana* flows, nerve impulses, and fluids in the body.

Breakfast is usually desirable. Hot foods and sweet and sour tastes. Reduce dry foods and bitter tastes. Warm or hot water and drinks. Raw nuts and nut butters. Spices: cinnamon, cardamom, cumin, ginger, cloves in moderation.

Vegetables	*Fruits*	*Grains*
cooked vegetables	sweet fruits	oats, cooked
asparagus	apricots	rice
beets	avocados	wheat
carrots	bananas	
cucumber	berries	————————
garlic	cherries	
green beans	coconut	No legumes
onions, cooked	fresh figs	except mung
sweet potato	grapefruit	beans, and black
radishes	lemons	and red lentils.
leafy greens	grapes	
in moderation	mangos	Oils: ghee and
	sweet melons	olive oil.
	sour oranges	
	papaya	
	peaches	
	sour fruits	

If your basic constitution is mixed (*vata-pitta* or *vata-kapha*), include portions for the second influential *dosha*.

Vata dosha is aggravated and increased during autumn and early winter. During these seasons all mind-body types can include some of the above foods and decrease others.

Mental and emotional peace and constructive lifestyle routines are important to restoring and maintaining balance.

A Food Plan to Balance Pitta Dosha

These guidelines can be used for *pitta* mind-body constitutions, to maintain *dosha* balance and to restore balance if necessary regardless of the basic constitution. *Pitta* influences digestion and metabolism, body temperature, and biological transformations.

Breakfast is usually all right. Avoid egg yolks, nuts, hot spices, honey, and hot drinks. Cool foods and drinks are better. Add sweet, bitter, and astringent tastes. Reduce use of sour tastes. Spices: black pepper, coriander, and cardamom.

Vegetables	*Fruits*	*Grains*
sweet and bitter vegetables	sweet fruits	basmati rice
asparagus	apples	oats, barley,
broccoli	avocado	wheat
brussels sprouts	figs	
cabbage	dark grapes	_____
cucumber	mangos	
cauliflower	melons	All legumes
celery	oranges	except lentils
green beans	pineapple	
leafy greens	plums	
peas	prunes	
parsley	raisins	
green peppers		
potato		
squash		

If your basic constitution is mixed (*pitta-vata* or *pitta-kapha*), to maintain balance, include smaller portions for the second *dosha*.

Pitta dosha is aggravated and increased during summer. During hot, dry seasons, all mind-body types can choose some of the above foods and decrease others.

Mental and emotional peace and constructive lifestyle routines are important to restoring and maintaining balance.

A Food Plan to Balance Kapha Dosha

These guidelines can be used for *kapha* mind-body constitutions, to maintain *dosha* balance, and to restore balance if necessary, regardless of the basic constitution. *Kapha* influences the heavy, moist aspects of the body.

Breakfast is usually not necessary. Avoid sugar, fats, dairy products, and salt. Ghee and oils only in small amounts. Choose light, dry foods. The main meal should be at the middle of the day, and only a light, dry meal in the evening. Avoid cold foods and drinks. Reduce use of sweet, sour, and salty tastes. Pungent, astringent, and bitter tastes are all right. All spices.

Vegetables	*Fruits*	*Grains*
pungent & bitter	apples	corn
vegetables	apricots	millet
asparagus	berries	oats, dry
beets	cherries	rye
broccoli	cranberries	barley
brussels sprouts	figs	basmati rice
cabbage	mangos	
cauliflower	peaches	————
celery	prunes	
eggplant	pomegranates	All legumes
garlic, onions		except kidney
peas		beans, soybeans
spinach		and black lentils
potato		

If your basic constitution is mixed (*kapha-pitta* or *kapha-vata*), include smaller portions for the second *dosha*.

Kapha dosha is aggravated and increased in the spring of the year. During this season, eat less and choose more dry, fibrous foods. During wet, cold seasons, all mind-body types can choose some of the above foods and decrease others.

Cultivate inner peace and exercise regularly.

Your Personal Application of
Life-Knowledge Program #3

1. Write a food selection plan for yourself for the pur-
    pose of restoring balance to your mind-body constitu-
    tion or for maintaining balance.

    _____

    _____

    _____

    _____

    _____

    _____

    _____

An Affirmation of Realization

At the innermost level of my being I am serenely peaceful.
I am completely fulfilled because soul-satisfied.
No longer blinded by delusions, I know what is true.
No longer confused by illusions, I see what is real.
Established in the Infinite, I live effectively
with flawless skill and easy grace.
I knowledgeably cooperate with the supportive laws
of nature and spontaneously demonstrate total wellness.

4

Routines for Mental
and Physical Cleansing

Unless we are always spiritually awake, mentally
alert, and in complete harmony with the actions of
nature, effective routines for cleansing and renewal of the
mind and body can be helpful at periodic intervals and
whenever we become aware of a need for them.

While engaged in wellness practices, we should know
that their ultimate purpose is to facilitate function and to
allow us, as spiritual beings, to efficiently express through
the mind and body. Our primary emphasis should be to
nurture spiritual awareness while attending to necessary
mental and physical activities. If, because of mental confusion or physical discomfort, spiritual growth is difficult
to actualize, as the mind is purified by intentional
endeavor and the body becomes healthier because of
adherence to regenerative routines, spiritual growth will
unfold more easily. A holistic approach to wellness requires
that we give attention to all levels of our being and to our
relationships with others and the environment.

To ensure spiritual integrity, be informed of the facts
of life, pray and meditate regularly, and train yourself to
be established in soul awareness at all times. Cultivate
the habit of soul-remembrance to avoid identification with
random thought processes, emotional states, invalid opinions of other people, and life-diminishing circumstances.
When established in soul awareness, we are calm and dis-

cerning. When not established in soul awareness, we may passively (or aggressively) be inclined to identify with outer conditions. One of the primary reasons for the problems many people have is that, because of feelings of loneliness, insecurity, or purposelessness, they tend to allow themselves to be attracted to and identified with outer conditions to the extent that awareness becomes clouded and the mind confused.

When clouded awareness and mental confusion prevail, intellectual errors mar understanding and prevent factual (truthful) discernment. Misperception (illusion) instead of accurate observation can occur. Behaviors may be impelled by moods, whims, blind habit, carelessness, or the impractical advice or personal influence of people with whom we associate. To return awareness to wholeness and think rationally and be soul-determined, a most helpful practice is to daily adhere to a self-care routine to enhance spiritual awareness, refresh the mind, and ensure physical well-being.

Because we cannot live effectively if we are dysfunctional, all restrictions to healthy, creative expression should be removed. A daily self-care routine for spiritual growth, mental acuity, and physical wellness is helpful for this purpose. One of the extra benefits of attending to a daily self-care routine is that it enhances our sense of purposefulness. When engaged in chosen activities we do something useful because we want to do so, instead of being compelled by subconscious conditionings to perform nonuseful actions or being pressured by demands or challenges from without. During the thirty minutes to one hour that we are devoted to our self-care practices, we are alone with our thoughts and our behaviors are determined by our own choices. The soul-empowerment we experience during our quiet time enables us to be decisive and focused during the remainder of the day.

For Mental Cleansing

Meditate regularly. When not meditating, maintain a constructive mental attitude. Cultivate optimism, cheerfulness, faith, and possibility-thinking. You can do it because you are a spiritual being with freedom to choose your mental states. Renounce pessimism, sadness or depression, uncertainty, and beliefs that challenging conditions of any kind are permanent. Expect (and allow) only constructive mental impulses to blossom into thoughts and imaginal states. Avoid destructive self-talk—the unregulated, negative mental conversations that may occur when attention is diffused or undisciplined. Learn to think rationally and use your powers of intelligence. Be open to intuitive insights and incidents of spontaneous discovery. A supportive aid to ordered thinking is to speak only constructive words with conscious intention. Purposeful, constructive actions are also supportive of ordered thinking.

Maintain an objective relationship to memories as mental records of prior perception and experience. View them as information only. Discern the difference between memories as information and emotions which may be associated with them. In this way, have access to memories without being unduly influenced by feelings of regret, sadness, anger, guilt, or hurt. Let memories of success and enjoyment remind you of life's goodness. If you remember past mistakes, let such memories motivate you to make wise choices now. Train yourself to live fully in the moment while looking to the future with optimism, curiosity, and purposefulness. Because you are a spiritual being, there is no need for you to be a victim of memories or to be restricted by self-defeating habits, conditioned mental states, or limiting beliefs.

Because many physical problems and difficulties which occur in the course of everyday living have a psychological basis, it is important to think rationally and to be emotionally balanced and mature. Our mental field comprises our awareness, the basis of perception and feeling; our sense of individuality, the basis of ego consciousness; the faculty of intelligence by which we discern; and the mind, which processes information. It is helpful, therefore, to remain as an objective witness to mental and emotional states rather than to become identified with them to the degree that we become soul-forgetful.

Helpful to ordering thought processes and balancing emotions is to live with intentional purpose. By doing what we know to be most useful, we learn to live successfully. New, constructive habits are then formed, emotions become coordinated with thoughts and actions, and success in endeavors improves our skills and increases our self-confidence. We awaken spiritually, become healthy-minded, and improve our functional abilities when we focus on essentials and disregard nonessentials. It is by right living that we prove to ourselves the actions and effects of the principles which determine and regulate all of life's processes. Having knowledge of how to live will not provide us the success and fulfillment we desire and deserve if we do not use it.

Effective Body Cleansing Routines

A daily self-care routine, common sense dietary regimens, and lifestyle practices which enable us to have harmonious relationships with nature and everyday events and circumstances contribute to maintaining a balance of the *doshas* which support our basic mind-body constitution. The body's immune system will then be strong, energy levels will be high, and keen interest in living will be pronounced. It is also important to avoid an accumulation of waste products and toxic matters due to *dosha* imbalance, inadequate digestion and assimilation of foods, or absorption of pollutants from the environment.

When the actions of the *doshas* are either excessive or deficient, corresponding symptoms can be observed. By the time symptoms are evident, *dosha* imbalance has progressed to the stage where discomfort or disease may manifest. The most useful approach to removing discomfort or disease is to reduce the symptoms of imbalance and restore the basic constitution to complete balance so that perfect health can be actualized. The mere absence of symptoms should not be considered a healthy condition. In the early stages of imbalance, *dosha* influences expand to regions of the body other than their natural sites or places of primary action. Symptoms of discomfort or impaired biological function may then follow.

A trained Ayurvedic physician can recognize which *doshas* and their influences are contributing to the patient-client's problem and recommend a specific therapeutic program to assist a return to healthy function. Because subtle causes of ailments may vary, similar superficial symptoms may have different causes and should be addressed. For instance, constipation may be caused by a *vata*, *pitta*, or *kapha* imbalance. If we know which *dosha* is excessive or deficient in influence, appropriate corrective action can be implemented to meet the precise need. One of the reasons why a therapeutic regimen is effective for one person but ineffective for others even though their symptoms may appear to be similar, is that underlying causes may differ. In this presentation of Ayurvedic principles and regimens I have chosen to focus on routines that balance the actions of the *doshas* rather than dwell on corrective regimens for specific symptoms. Special needs should be addressed by a knowledgeable, trained practitioner of life-knowledge.

Vata dosha may be aggravated by excesses of any kind: too much eating, fasting, talking, frantic movement, exertion, suppression of natural urges, sleeplessness, and worry. Too much food which is bitter, pungent, dry, or light can cause *vata* imbalance, as can cold and rainy seasons when the weather is cloudy and stormy. This *dosha* may also be somewhat disturbed after digestion has been completed. Old age is usually the stage of one's life when *vata dosha* influences are normally excessive.

Some symptoms of disturbed vata dosha influences are thirst, shaking, dryness, yawning, melancholy, erratic thinking and behaviors, mental confusion, emotional instability, and pain in various parts of the body. In instances of severe *dosha* disturbance it is important to determine whether symptoms are due to excessive *dosha* influence or to a blockage or diminishing of influences.

Pitta dosha may be aggravated by anger, grief, physical exertion, impaired powers of digestion, excessive use of foods which are bitter, acid, salty, or dry, and excessive exposure to sunlight and heat. It tends to be aggravated in summer and early autumn, at noon and midnight, and its influence is stronger during middle age.

Some symptoms of disturbed pitta dosha influences are stomach acidity, fainting, restlessness, thirst, desire for cooling influences, delirium, hysteria, excessive perspiration, and acrid body odor.

Kapha dosha may be aggravated by a sedentary lifestyle, and by excessive use of sweet, acid, salty, oily, or heavy foods. It is aggravated during winter and spring seasons, and its influence is stronger during childhood.

Some symptoms of disturbed kapha dosha influences are heaviness, drowsiness, nausea, aversion to food, tiredness, and a feeling that one is slowing down or getting old too soon. There may also be an increase of mucus and other thick, moist substances in the body, and evidence of the body's attempts to eliminate them.

The way to correct *dosha* imbalance and a need for mental and physical cleansing is to adopt appropriate mental attitudes, personal behaviors, and regular lifestyle regimens which are supportive of our purposes.

The Dietary Way to Balance the Doshas

Choose foods which do not excessively increase any of the doshas while including all six tastes at the major meal of the day (see chapter 3 for guidelines).

To cleanse the body, for one or more weeks choose a balanced diet of complex carbohydrates, legumes, vegetables, and fruits. Avoid dairy products, heavy or oily foods, and all commercially processed foods. During this program, frequently drink modest amounts of distilled water, to flush waste products from the body's systems.

Exercise regularly. Brisk walking and swimming are good forms of exercise. A daily hatha yoga routine can be helpful for improving muscle tone, stretching, and encouraging blood and lymph circulation and balanced flows of life force. T'ai Chi is excellent for centering, balancing *prana* flows, and improving attunement with the rhythms of nature.

Have a regular sleep schedule. Go to bed early and awaken early to attend to your morning self-care and meditation routine.

To keep the skin clean, bathe daily. During this cleansing program, before bathing brush the skin with a dry towel and massage the entire body with a small quantity of warm sesame oil (described later in this chapter).

A complete fast is not usually recommended. For body cleansing for one or a few days, drink only freshly made fruit and vegetable juices. Use fruit juices until noon for their cleansing effect, and fresh vegetable juices (carrots, beets, spinach, celery—with perhaps a modest portion of onion or garlic) during the afternoon hours. Dilute fruit juices with pure water. Fruit and vegetable juices provide nutrients and have a cleansing effect. A less extreme regimen is to eat fresh fruits until noon and vegetable soup in the afternoon and evening.

To make vegetable soup, simmer cubed potatoes, tomatoes, carrots, green vegetables, onions, garlic, and other vegetables desired, for thirty minutes.

For a substantial meal, useful for physical cleansing and for balancing all three *doshas*, the following recipe has been found to be helpful:

 1 cup lentils or split mung beans
 1 cup basmati rice
 1 inch fresh ginger, peeled and finely chopped
 1 small handful fresh cilantro leaves (or fresh spinach)
1/2 cup water
 1 tablespoon ghee (clarified butter)
 1 inch cinnamon stick
 3 cardamom pods, remove and use seeds
 5 whole cloves, crushed
10 black peppercorns
 3 bay leaves
1/4 teaspoon turmeric
 6 cups water

Wash lentils and soak in water for a few hours. Wash rice. Blend ginger, cilantro and 1/2 cup of water until liquefied. Crush the cloves, cardamom seeds, and peppercorns.

Add cinnamon, cloves, cardamom, peppercorns, and bay leaves to ghee in a saucepan, on medium heat. Stir until the fragrance is discernible. Add blended items and the turmeric. Stir until lightly brown.

Stir in the rice and lentils or beans. Pour in the 6 cups of water. Bring to a boil and simmer for 5 minutes. Cover and turn heat to very low for 15 minutes.

This meal is nourishing and easy to digest. The spices improve digestive fire and beneficially influence the *doshas*.

Optional: Include sliced or cubed vegetables of your choice at boiling and simmering stage.

How to Make Ghee (clarified butter)

Heat one pound of unsalted butter in a heavy pot over medium heat until it simmers. Froth will rise to the surface. Turn heat to low. The liquid butter will turn a golden yellow color. Solids will sink to the bottom. When a drop of water thrown into the ghee produces a crackling sound, remove from heat. Allow to cool for several minutes before straining through cheesecloth or any clean cloth. Ghee can be stored at room temperature or refrigerated. Only a small quantity is needed as a cooking oil.

Herbal Supplementation

Garlic is a useful herb for body cleansing. Many people claim immunity from cold and flu viruses because of regular garlic use. Although garlic capsules without the characteristic odor are now on the market, I prefer to use fresh garlic. This herb has hot, bitter, and pungent tastes. It is considered to be good for rejuvenation purposes and enlivens powers of digestion. It helps to reduce symptoms of excess *vata* influences and increases *pitta* influences. The warming effect of garlic is useful during rainy seasons and winter. Fresh garlic can be thinly sliced or crushed for salads and cooked foods or sandwiches.

An herbal compound used for centuries in Asia and becoming more popular in the West is *Chyavan Prash* (the spelling varies from one manufacturer to another, as may the ingredients). The common base is fresh amla fruit (said to have more than one thousand times the Vitamin C content of an equal portion of fresh oranges). Herbs such as ashwaganda, shatavari, cardamom, cinnamon leaf, long pepper, and others, are added, along with ghee, natural sugar, and sometimes honey as "vehicles" to transport the herbal essences to the tissues. A teaspoonful is usually taken once or twice a day, on an empty stomach, followed by a small portion of warm milk or water to aid assimilation. Herbs have a subtle effect and require regular usage over a period of time for maximum benefits. Pregnant women and people with diabetes should consult their physician before using this product.

According to folk legend, Chyavan was an elderly sage whose health was restored to radiant fitness by the regular ingestion of this *prash* (herbal food). If you live in or near a city or town with a sizable Indian community, you may want to visit one of their food stores and ask for this product. It is commonly available, usually imported from India although some companies in the United States are now producing it.

Nasal Cleansing

Some of the functions of the nose are to filter moisture, warm the air that is inhaled, respond to smells, create mucus, allow sinus drainage, and affect the nervous system. The external part of the nose gathers air that is inhaled to the internal regions. The inner walls of the nasal cavity have convoluted structures that stir and circulate air and mix it with moisture. When we exhale, moist air rewarms and moistens the lining of the nose that was somewhat dried by the inhaled air.

The nasal lining is covered with a membrane that secretes mucus. Here, dust is collected, along with bacteria, viruses, fungi, and other small particles which might be present in the air we breathe. The mucus that is produced moves upward and backward towards the throat where it is swallowed, and it and any potentially harmful microbes are dissolved by digestive enzymes in the intestinal tract. The movement of this blanket of mucus is made possible by the constant motion of millions of hair-like structures (*cilia*) growing out of the mucus lining.

Sometimes, however, the mucus in the nose is too thick, becomes dry, and adheres to the cilia and mucus lining. Crusts can then build up, providing a home for microbes such as those which cause the common cold. The opposite condition occurs when the mucus is too liquid and causes watery dripping.

Mucus is both produced and secreted in various parts of the body. It is excreted or expelled through the skin, kidneys, bowels, and lungs when it is excessive. Improper diet can contribute to excess mucus that has to be excreted. For many people, too much use of milk and some starchy foods will create excess mucus.

Small passageways from the sinus to the nasal cavity allow the sinuses to drain. When these become obstructed and free circulation of air and mucus flows is impeded, the sinuses begin to absorb air and a partial vacuum is created. Mucus, blood, and tissue fluids can then accumulate, creating irritation, pressure, and pain. This condition, sinusitis, is often accompanied by headaches.

The nasal cavity can be cleansed by flushing with a mild, warm salt water solution. Nature provides small quantities of saline solution in the form of tears that drain from the eyes into the nasal cavity through the lacrimal ducts, so using a salt water solution for cleansing is a natural, beneficial procedure. Being able to breathe freely is supportive of our physical and psychological well-being because of the relationship between breathing and flows of life force in the body.

Stir one-quarter teaspoon of salt and one cup of body temperature water in a container to be used for nasal cleansing. The container should have a spout that enables you to pour the water into the nostrils.

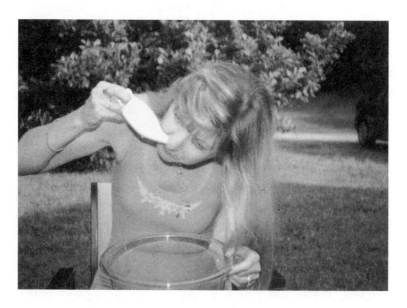

Bend forward over a sink, tilting your head slightly to one side. Into the uppermost nostril, insert the spout of the container and let the water flow. It will flow out of the nostril on the opposite side. When the container is empty, refill with salt water solution and repeat the process from the other side. When finished, gently blow through both nostrils. While doing this procedure you can breathe easily through your open mouth. Nasal cleansing removes dry or thick mucus and moisturizes the nasal cavity.

This procedure can be done anytime its need becomes obvious to you. Many people find it especially helpful during excessively dry seasons of the year and when dust and pollen are in the air.

Cleansing the Subtle Channels
Through Which Life Force Flows

A useful *pranayama* for cleansing the subtle channels (*nadis*) can be practiced as part of your morning self-care routine or just before meditation practice.

Life forces (*prana*) are constantly circulating through the subtle astral sheath, the vehicle which interpenetrates the physical body. Two main currents flow along the spinal pathway. The force through the left channel is stronger when air flows more obviously through the left nostril. This is called the Moon or lunar breath. It is stronger through the right channel when air flows more obviously through the right nostril. This is called the Sun or solar breath. When we are psychologically and physically healthy, the lunar current is dominant for about two hours, followed by a two-hour phase of solar current dominance. When the lunar current is dominant, there is a slight swelling of the erectile tissues in the right nasal passageway, which partially blocks the air flow during inhalation. When the solar current is dominant, the tissues in the right nasal passageway shrink and the tissues in the left nasal passageway are enlarged.

During the lunar current phase, the right hemisphere of the brain is more active, inclining one to be more introspective and subjective. When the solar current is more dominant, the left hemisphere of the brain is more active, inclining one to be more outward, goal-directed, and intentional in objective involvements. During the transition phases, one may become aware of changes in moods and behavioral inclinations.

Ayurvedic texts recommend encouraging right nostril

(solar-heating) breathing when involved in executive actions requiring decision-making and accomplishing projects, and at mealtime. Digestive fire is naturally stronger then. Left nostril breathing (lunar-cooling) is suitable for calming the emotions, creative thinking, using imagination, and restful sleep. Sleeping on the left side, for instance, tends to cause partial closing of the left nostril and encourages solar breathing, which warms the body. Sleeping on the right side causes partial closing of the right nostril and encourages lunar breathing, which is ideal for dreamless sleep.

When we are emotionally disturbed or physically unwell, the normal two-hour, lunar-solar phases do not always occur as they should. Either right or left nostril breathing may be dominant. To restore or to maintain a balance of flows of *prana*, alternate nostril breathing can be intentionally practiced.

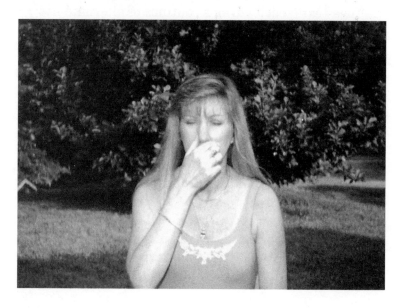

1. Sit upright and relaxed. Put your hand to your nose, close one nostril with your finger or thumb and gently inhale. Do this with the other nostril, also, to determine the one through which the air is more freely flowing.

2. Close the nostril through which the air flow is diminished. Inhale smoothly (and a little more deeply than usual but not excessively so) through the open nostril. Pause for a fleeting moment. Close that nostril and exhale smoothly through the other one. Pause a moment, and repeat the procedure in reverse. If you start with the right nostril: inhale through it, pause, exhale through the left nostril, pause, inhale through the left nostril, pause, exhale through the right nostril. Do this three times. Breathe in and out through both nostrils three times. Repeat the entire sequence three times.

Yoga texts teach various routines of alternate nostril breathing for specific purposes. The one described here is the most basic practice and is ideal for encouraging psychological and physical balance.

Bowel Cleansing

It is important to have regular, complete bowel movements. If fiber is lacking in the diet, it can be supplemented by selecting more foods with fiber and adding wheat or oat bran to grain recipes. For special purposes, when needed, psyllium husk in powdered form can be taken: one teaspoonful, or more, stirred in a glass of water, once or twice a day. It will attract moisture to the large intestine and add bulk. Psyllium husk powder is available in most drug stores, usually flavored and sweetened. It would be better to obtain the natural product from your local health food store.

From time to time, when necessary, a warm water enema may be used to encourage complete cleansing.

How to Apply a Warm Oil Massage

Massaging the skin with warm oil soothes the nervous and endocrine systems and balances all three *dosha* influences, especially *vata*. Sesame oil is ideal for general use. Start by warming one-fourth cup of the oil. Place a cup or plastic bottle containing the oil in a larger bowl or pan of medium hot water for a few minutes.

Use the palm of the hand and open fingers to massage your entire body, with circular motions over the joints and straight movements for the neck, shoulders, back, chest, arms, and legs. You may thinly coat the entire body with oil at the beginning, to let it soak the skin.

Use light to moderate pressure when stroking. Start with your head, massaging the scalp, face, and ears. (Scalp massage can be done only every few days if washing your hair every day is an inconvenience.)

Move down to your neck and upper back, then shoulders, upper arms, forearms, and hands. Use a gentle, circular motion over your heart and abdomen. Massage your back as far as you can reach. The legs can be massaged more vigorously. Spend more time working on your ankles and tops and bottoms of your feet. If you feel mild pain when you probe your ankles and feet with your fingers, continue until the feeling of discomfort is reduced. There are reflex centers in the feet which correspond to organs and glands in the body which are beneficially affected by gentle foot massage.

It is a good idea to have a towel or small rug (to be used only for this purpose) to place on the bathroom floor, to catch any dripping oil. Sit on a stool or on the commode seat when massaging the lower legs and feet. The entire process can be completed in a few minutes, after which the oil can be washed off with a warm shower. Wipe your feet well before stepping into the shower, to prevent slipping. It may require practice to learn to accomplish this routine without using too much oil. When laundering the towels which have oily residue, it is better to do them separately. If any oil remains in the towel fibers, it may be a good idea to hang them to dry rather than dry them in a hot clothes dryer, because oils are flammable.

Open Yourself Completely to the Rhythms and Flows of the Supportive, Nurturing Currents of the Universe

Because the One Consciousness exists, all that is in manifestation is an expression of it. When we are in harmony with the rhythms and flows of the universe, its supportive currents nurture our well-being and effortlessly provide our every need. The great essential is for us to learn to be open to life so that its actions and influences can spontaneously express through and around us.

We can help ourselves be more open and responsive by maintaining right Self-understanding, expanding our awareness, and living so that affluence (being in the flow of nurturing influences and of resources) is our normal experience. Whenever we are aware of any restrictions that cloud our awareness or interfere with mental, physical, or circumstantial harmony, we can by practical means remove those restrictions. Knowledge of the processes of life enables us to effectively participate with them so that we experience fulfillment while we also make useful contributions to the spiritual, mental, physical, social, and environmental well-being of others with whom we share our present time-space sojourn.

We are in this world for a higher purpose than to only live in comfort for a few decades. We are here to awaken to the fact that we are agents of the Higher Power which is ever impelling souls to awaken to illumination of consciousness. We live in an era of rapid, transformative activity which is resulting in mass spiritual awakening and a need to examine social, economic, political, and ecological issues which affect the planet and its inhabitants. As we become more conscious and functional, we can be more effective in relating to events and circumstances.

The important matter is for us to grow to spiritual, mental, and emotional maturity. This requires that we be willing to awaken from conditioned self-conscious (egocentric) states to awareness of our spiritual potential. Since all of the practices and routines we learn and use to enhance wellness and function are for the purpose of freeing us to live effectively, we should be aware of the fact that radiant health and functional skills should serve our higher purposes. We should not desire better health and more knowledge only to satisfy small-minded desires or to perpetuate behaviors and relationships which restrict spiritual impulses. We should, instead, expand awareness so that our innate knowledge (which includes knowledge of God and all of life's processes) is completely unfolded.

When it is, we are fully enlightened: free, with no restricting influences to prevent our grace-directed actions.

We can prepare ourselves to be responsive to the impulses of grace by doing what we can to remove restrictions that block its flow. At the soul level we can remain stable in Self-understanding and aspire to further awakening. At the mental level we can cultivate intellectual skills and rational thinking. At the emotional level we can choose maturity over immaturity. At the physical level we can nurture radiant wellness. In endeavors we can perform constructive actions. In relationships we can be caring and supportive. Because of our prudent endeavors and God's enlivening and redemptive grace, we can be assured that optimal unfoldments on all levels will be actualized and that our soul destiny will be fulfilled.

It is helpful to remember that, because we are individualized expressions of God's consciousness, our role in awakening to the full potential is to remove or renounce all beliefs, mental attitudes, behaviors, and conditions which in any way restrict or suppress the impulses of our divine nature to flow.

Many sincere devotees, although faithful in their studies and their daily prayer and meditation routines, do not experience satisfying spiritual growth because of one or a number of reasons. They may be attached to invalid opinions or beliefs, habitually err in perceptions, prefer to be emotionally immature, disregard basic health practices, or resist opportunities to learn how to live well. Some devotees have mental conflicts about whether or not it is permissible for them to want to live well in this world. They may be afraid to live well because they do not yet know how, may mistakenly think that enjoyable living in this world is incompatible with their aspiration for spiritual growth, or may have experienced failure and misfortune. They are wise not to want to be blindly or self-centeredly involved, but they need to realize that here and now is the only opportunity they have to learn to live correctly. They need to learn to open themselves to life.

By living with enlightened (knowledgeable) understanding while the opportunity to do so is available, we become capable of living freely now and in the future. The universe is a play of cosmic forces with origins in God's consciousness, and we are expressive units of God's consciousness. Awakening to this realization is liberating. We are supposed to be knowledgeable, healthy, functional, and affluent. If we are not actualizing our potential, we are denying our spiritual reality and suppressing our innate urge to have awareness restored to wholeness. Learn to live consciously and well. Be happy. Be thankful.

Speak this Affirmation

I am happy to be alive. I am thankful to know my true nature and relationship with God and God's universe.
I rejoice to awaken to knowledge of how to live effectively and I do so with skillful diligence. I am ever open and responsive to the nurturing impulses and actions of life.

Rest in Absolute Peace of Soul

Below the threshold of your thoughts and feelings, at the level from which impulses arise, you are firmly established in the reality of pure, conscious being. Here, absolute peace prevails because wholeness is the permanent condition of the soul.

Turn your attention to this level during interludes of surrendered meditation. It does not have to be cultivated or created, for it ever exists as it is. When the random movements which ordinarily occur in your field of awareness are stilled, peace of soul is naturally experienced. Let enjoyment at this level of your being be permanent while you are engaged in activities and relationships.

When you are established in peace of soul, entirely beneficial effects occur at mental and physical levels. Healing influences arise from the field of pure consciousness to balance mind-body processes. The emotional nature is calmed. The mind is cleansed. The intellect is purified. Self-centeredness is dissolved. Powers of perception are improved. Effortless, harmonious relationships with life's processes are experienced. Supportive circumstances and events appropriately unfold. While you are attending to necessary matters, behind all of your thoughts and actions, soul peace remains your anchor, your resting place, your permanent abode.

Having known these things [the principles of Ayurveda], the [ancient] sages applied them and experienced optimum well-being and untiring long life.
– *Charaka Samhita* –

Your Personal Application of
Life-Knowledge Program #4

1. For mental and physical cleansing, review this chapter and write your specific routines.

_____

_____

_____

_____

_____

_____

_____

_____

An Affirmation of Commitment

Ever soul-centered and open to learning and growth,
I utilize all practical means to facilitate radiant health,
functional efficiency, success in all actions, and
satisfying, authentic spiritual growth.

5

Rejuvenation, Enlightened Living, and Conscious Immortality

There is nothing mysterious or magical about the causative laws that determine our ability to actualize total wellness and flawless spiritual awareness. They can be easily learned by anyone who is reasonably intelligent, sufficiently open-minded, and curious enough to experiment with them.

The soul has a persistent drive to prevail over circumstances. When its attention is outwardly directed, it is inclined to accomplish its purposes even when confronted by what may seem to be insurmountable obstacles; thus the instances of dramatic healings, heroic behaviors, and successful endeavors to achieve idealized goals which are sometimes publicized in secular media. When the soul's attention flows back to its source, it is impelled by an urge to have awareness returned to wholeness with such constancy that spiritual growth occurs, resulting in spontaneous unfoldment of its innate qualities.

Healthy-minded people naturally desire to be aware, vital, and happy. Also, either because of their aversion to death or intuitive knowledge of their immortality, they want to live forever. Because souls are as immortal as God is, forever-life is already being experienced whether we are aware of this fact or not. Some ill, confused, or dysfunctional people are tired, apathetic, and hope for death or unconsciousness as a way to be released from their troubles. What they may not know, is that if they do succumb to unconsciousness, after a duration of rest their attention will again turn to the sense-perceived realms and their learning and growing experiences will continue.

Since we have to live, why not learn to live in the best way possible? Why not be healthy, functional, mentally competent, and successful? Why not live with enlightened (knowledgeable) understanding? Why not be completely Self-realized and God-conscious? All of these fulfillments can be actualized while we are embodied.

Chronically dysfunctional and problem-centered people usually believe their circumstances to have external causes. What is needed is an adjustment of perspective: from believing that one is a victim of existing conditions to envisioning limitless possibilities from the vantage point of soul-identity perception. Since we are incarnated Spirit-mind-body beings, our spiritual awareness is superior to mental and physical states. We need to learn to unfold and effectively use our spiritual abilities.

Confronting the Facts of Life and Introducing Constructive Influences

Since we cannot choose different ancestors, we have to do the best we can with the genetic characteristics and basic mind-body constitution with which we were born. Nor can we do anything about the environmental circumstances provided us when we were children, completely control the forces of nature, prevent the planet from undergoing changes caused by shifting land masses, or immediately change the thinking and behaviors of others which influence social, political, and economic conditions. However, when we arrive at the stage where we are capable of self-determination, we are free to choose our thoughts, moods, relationships, goals, and behaviors. What we have already experienced has been, for the most part, the result of our own states of consciousness, mental states, choices, and behaviors. Knowing this, we must admit that most of the illnesses, grievances, and problems that people have are consciously or unconsciously self-created or agreed to. By accepting this idea—or by considering it as a possibility if we are not yet able to believe it—we can experiment with our thoughts and behaviors to see whether or not we can introduce useful change into our lives when necessary or desired, rid ourselves of restrictive circumstances, experience a supportive relationship with nature, and more obviously unfold our innate potential.

Most of the causes of premature physical death are preventable. The three major causes of physical demise in industrially developed regions of the world are heart disease, stroke, and cancer, followed by pneumonia, influenza, bronchitis, accidents, diabetes, arteriosclerosis, and liver disease. Among young people with heart disease, the causes are usually congenital or rheumatic. Beyond age forty-five, arteriosclerosis of the heart's blood vessels is usually the underlying cause. Elevated blood cholesterol is a factor in causing arteriosclerosis, and this condition is directly related to improper diet. A stroke occurs when blood flow to the brain is blocked because of clogged arteries secondary to arteriosclerosis or a rupture of blood vessels due to high blood pressure, or a combination of these conditions. In cultures where food intake is low in calories and rich in nutritive qualities, the incidence of heart disease and cancer is much lower than in cultures where excess protein (usually meat), high fat, and a nutrition-deficient diet are routinely chosen. It is not surprising that, in regions of the world where use of "fast foods" and meat and dairy products has been encouraged, the incidence of diseases common in affluent regions where dietary improprieties and excesses are common is increasing. Lifestyle changes are also a contributing factor. In economically developing regions of the world, the pace of living has generally increased, along with stress and a variety of psychological complications.

By confronting, examining, and understanding the causes of conditions that determine effects, we can introduce constructive influences when necessary. When we are not aware of the facts, we may be at the mercy of circumstances beyond our ability to regulate. When we are aware of them but choose not to do anything to help ourselves or to replace oppressive conditions, unfortunate consequences that manifest are due to our negligence. When we are adequately informed, emotionally mature, and willing to be responsible for our actions, we can enter into a harmonious relationship with nature and have its complete support. In many instances, by attitude adjustment and behavior modification, along with dietary changes and implementation of life-enhancing regimens, the progress of physical deterioration can be stopped and a return to wellness can be demonstrated.

The realm of nature includes all manifesting aspects and actions of God's Consciousness: the field of primordial nature, Universal Mind, causal (magnetic-electric) influences, astral (life force) characteristics, and physical substances. If we endeavor to implement desired changes by working at the physical level only, our efforts will be but marginally successful. The Ayurvedic approach to restoring and maintaining health takes into consideration the most subtle levels at which life expresses.

Facilitate Spiritual Awakening and Growth as Your Primary Approach to Total Wellness

Nurture spiritual awareness by acquiring accurate information about the reality and characteristics of God, what primordial nature is (as an objective expression of God's creative energy), the categories of cosmic manifestation, what souls are and how they become involved with mind and matter, and how to facilitate the processes of soul awakening and unfoldment. One of the reasons why many people are not successful in accomplishing their purposes is that they are not adequately informed about these fundamental matters. They prefer to live superficially, to barely survive, hoping they will be fortunate enough to experience reasonably comfortable old age and a painless death. When they have a major problem, they hope someone else will provide the solution.

As a soul, you are a unit of the One Consciousness. When you are established in realization (conscious knowledge and experience) of your essential nature, you are at peace within yourself because Self-complete, and your awareness is no longer fragmented or divided. When you are not established in realization of your essential nature, your awareness tends to identify with mental processes and sensory urges. Self-knowledge removes soul awareness from distracting influences. It is realized as a result of intellectual and intuitive examination of your real nature and awakening to actual experience of it. The life-knowledge way to wholeness and personal fulfillment is based on an understanding of spiritual realities, and all of the recommended procedures are helpful to balancing the physical and mental systems so that spiritual awareness can unfold easily and naturally.

Learn to Relate Harmoniously to Universal Mind—the Mind of God

Our mind which processes perceptions and information is a particularized unit of Universal Mind energized by soul force. Our awareness interacts with Universal Mind, which is responsive to our mental states, thoughts, imagery, and desires. Because the principle of mental correspondences is causative and impersonal, it produces conditions and circumstances in our lives regardless of whether or not our mental states are constructive. We should, therefore, regulate physical and mental impulses, mental attitudes, thought processes, imaginative states, and desires, so that only entirely constructive, life-enhancing results are manifested.

The most effective way to adjust mental states and organize thought processes is to cultivate spiritual awareness and synchronize behaviors, emotional states, and thinking. It is often easier to act and feel our way into a constructive mental state than it is to control thoughts by will power alone. This is why spiritual practices are emphasized along with intentional, purposeful actions and regulation of emotional states.

Avoid verbalizing self-defeating thoughts. Even when

you do not feel happy or confident, avoid affirming unhappiness or feelings of insecurity. Never say anything about yourself, others, or circumstances, that you do not want to have manifested. Never say, "I'm no good," "I have no confidence," "I'm lonely," "No one loves me," "I can't," "I'm incurably ill," "I'm poor, and always will be," "I'll never accomplish anything worthwhile," "I'm an addict and always will be," or any other self-limiting words. If you must say something, say:

- "I am a spiritual being, innately endowed with the qualities, capacities, and knowledge of God."
- "Established in soul awareness and in harmonious accord with life's processes, I am confident."
- "I am established in wholeness."
- "I can choose to do whatever needs to be done."
- "God, through and as me, can easily and flawlessly accomplish all worthwhile purposes."
- "I acknowledge the innate divinity of every person, and all my relationships are supportive."
- "Wholeness is my true condition; any appearance to the contrary must be harmonized or dissolved."
- "I am affluent, in the flow of limitless resources."
- "I am a free, spiritual being—without attachments, addictions, or limitations of any kind."

My guru, Paramahansa Yogananda, told disciples: "When your body needs rest, provide it opportunity to rest—but never say or believe that *you* are tired, because *you* as spirit cannot be tired." On another occasion, he said, "I never allow the word 'impossible' to take root in my mind; nor should you."

Train yourself to use your powers of creative imagination to *visualize*, *believe*, and *feel* the reality of ideal circumstances for yourself and others. Regularly engage in possibility-thinking by mentally and intuitively seeing and knowing what can be true for you. Do this with gentle, relaxed attention, knowing yourself to be grounded in the Infinite, in harmonious relationship with the actions of Universal Mind which spontaneously and appropriately unfolds circumstances and events to meet your every need. It is life's inclination (some refer to this as "God's will") to fulfill purposes. When you are in harmony with life's purpose-fulfilling inclinations, the Power that enlivens the universe and directs its processes will be expressive through and around you.

Become Aware of and Live From the Level of Causal Influences

Magnetic and electric forces in nature are responsive to states of consciousness and mental states. The patterns corresponding to the faculties of hearing, touch, sight, smell, and taste, and the organs of speech, movement, dexterity, elimination, and reproduction, along with the various aspects of the mental field, comprise your causal body which interpenetrates your astral and physical bodies. The mental faculties and causal organs of the senses of action are produced by the actions of the attributes (*gunas*) of Consciousness as they express at mental and causal levels. The empowering, intelligently directed forces that express as these attributes are the determining actions of the governing influences: *vata* (ether-air influence); *pitta* (fire-water influence); and *kapha* (water-earth influence). These actions in our mind and body are regulated by our states of consciousness, mental states, emotional states, foods, behaviors, and environmental factors. This is why the Ayurvedic approach to wellness and function is holistic: it includes everything which is supportive of us and our constructive purposes.

Learn to be aware at deeper levels than the physical. Be aware of your vital forces at the astral level and of the subtle counterparts of the organs of sense perception and actions at the causal level. Know that you, as the soul, are the immortal, formless being perceiving through the senses and moving through the body. Instead of being dependent upon the organs of senses and of actions, let them be responsive to your intentions and needs. In this way, cultivate your powers of extrasensory perception and allow exceptional abilities to express.

Balance Your Vital Forces

When you are soul-centered, your vital forces are naturally balanced; when they are not, nurture Self-knowledge and mental and emotional calm. Train yourself to always be soul-centered, aware, observant, and even-minded. Avoid stress; ensure sufficient rest and sleep; avoid worry, anxiety, and restlessness. Conserve your vital forces and increase their quantity and quality. Surplus vital forces are transmuted into a finer vital essence (*ojas*), which strengthens the body's immune system, manifests as the radiance of health, refines the astral or vital body, and energizes the mind. Be established in soul awareness, with clear understanding and with mastery of sensory and mental impulses. You *can* do this.

Exercise regularly in accord with your wisdom-led inclinations and your basic mind-body constitution. For *vata* constitutions, exercise should be moderate because strenuous, frantic exercise tends to aggravate and increase *vata* characteristics. For *pitta* constitutions, exercise should be vitalizing but not competitive because intensity tends to aggravate and increase *pitta* characteristics. For *kapha* constitutions, exercise should be more vigorous and sustained, to overcome inertia and heaviness which is characteristic of *kapha dosha* influences. The best way to exercise is to do so until you feel vitalized and happy, rather than exert too much effort or feel that you have to struggle to accomplish a goal.

In special instances, chiropractic adjustments or other intentional bodywork such as acupressure and deep massage can be helpful for the purpose of removing obstructions to the flow of vital forces.

Wisely Use Available Physical Resources

Regulate your lifestyle routines to balance activity and rest. Nature thrives on regularity. Awaken early, before dawn, to attend to personal self-care routines and meditation practice. Have your meals on a regular schedule. Have regular work hours and scheduled times for relaxation and recreation. Learn by practice to synchronize your activities with the flows of nature so that you have its full support and live effortlessly. When you are out of harmony with nature, when circumstances are too challenging, when you are overstressed or struggling, analyze your mental and emotional states and your motives and behaviors, and make adjustments to restore balance.

A key to healthy, long life is to habitually choose to consume only the amount of food needed and no more. Consuming excess food depletes the body's vital forces because of the extra work required to process and eliminate what is not immediately needed and the waste products which may accumulate. Ayurvedic texts recommend that the maximum quantity of food taken at one meal to be that which can be held in the cupped palms of both hands. The ideal is to have a sufficient quantity with emphasis on quality. Foods should be nutrition-rich, chosen to balance and support the mind-body constitution.

Controlled studies with white mice, and with a few other animals, indicate that a low-calorie, nutrition-rich diet contributes to improved health, lower incidence of disease, and a longer vital, active life span. There is no reason to suppose that results of such a diet plan are not equally beneficial for human beings. In fact, research along these lines has already been done, and is ongoing.

Dr. Roy L. Walford, a professor of pathology at the UCLA School of Medicine in Los Angeles, California, and a delegate to a White House Conference on Aging, has written about his findings in scores of scientific articles and several books. Two of his books are *Maximum Lifespan* and *The Anti-Aging Plan*. In the latter book he wrote of the results experienced by himself and five others of a research team who lived together in Biosphere 2, a project established in southern Arizona to determine how effectively human beings could live in a self-contained, life-supporting environment closed off from contact with the outside atmosphere. Inside the man-made facility, which covered only a few acres of land, the residents grew their food and recycled their wastes. Over 3,800 carefully selected species of plants and animals were tended and observed. As a physician and researcher, Dr. Walford supervised the meals for the residents of Biosphere 2. A few published details indicate some of the results.

The average value of blood cholesterol of the residents before starting the project was 191. Six months later the average cholesterol value was 123. The starting average blood pressure was 110 over 75. After a few months, the average blood pressure was 90 over 58. The skin of two of the residents who had severe facial acne before starting the project cleared rapidly as a result of their new diet. All of the residents were in better health, had more energy, and had lost their excess body weight.

The low-calorie, nutrition-rich food plan is not a starvation diet. It is low in fats and high in complex carbohydrates and a variety of colorful vegetables, with some fruit. Protein needs are usually easily met on a vegetarian diet by choosing a variety of foods, being sure to have beans or other legumes at the same meal with grains such as brown rice or corn. The combination of beans and grains provides a balance of amino acids so that protein requirements for replenishing body cells are met. The average person needs only a daily portion of approximately two ounces of a protein-rich food. Excessive protein intake works a hardship on the body.

Establish and maintain supportive relationships. See to your relationship with God first, by cultivating spiritual growth and learning to be established in Self-knowledge. Nurture mental and spiritual attunement with your spiritual teachers or mentors. Adhere to a regular schedule of right living with spiritual practices as your foundation. Learn to be on "friendly terms with a friendly world," knowing that the universe is supportive of you. Maintain respectful, supportive relationships with people with whom you live and work, and with friends and associates of your larger social circle. Cultivate friendly relations with all living things and creatures. Practice harmlessness, truthfulness, and honesty in all relationships.

Provide a comfortable and secure home for yourself, and for members of your family if you have that responsibility. Make your abode a sanctuary. Keep it comfortable, clean, orderly, and secure. Cultivate the habit of removing your shoes when entering your house, to keep the floors and carpets clean and uncontaminated. While you are inwardly anchored in the Infinite, your body dwells on earth; provide a supportive environment for its wellbeing and comfort. If possible, have a room or a private place set aside to meditate. With your home as your base, you can go forth to attend to your duties and activities and return for rest and refreshment. When you are physically secure, you are free to nurture your mind and soul and to accomplish worthwhile purposes.

Be wise and prudent when using physical resources, including money. Because we are on earth for but a few decades, nothing belongs to us; we have only the temporary use of physical resources. Use resources wisely, without grasping at things or circumstances, and without waste. Money is a convenient medium of exchange; with it we can obtain other things and pay for services rendered. Know it for what it is, and handle it skillfully. Open channels through which money and resources can flow to you by first opening your mind and awareness to the idea of affluence, and then by doing whatever practical things you can do to earn or attract money and resources.

Remember that everything flows to you from the Source regardless of the outer form of your provision or supply. Knowing this, trust the Source for everything while doing your practical best to be self-responsible for your well-being. Manage your resources carefully. Think about abundance instead of lack. If you have a regular income, save an agreed-upon percentage to prudently invest, apportion a percentage for good works, pay bills on time, avoid impulsive buying, maintain a surplus in your bank account, purchase quality items which are durable and serviceable. Know yourself to be in partnership with a Life and a Purpose larger than you are.

Know everything around you to be a manifestation of the creative energy of God. Say, "Wherever I look, I see God." Of course, the outer appearance-realm is not the totality of God, but it is a dramatization of God's cosmic forces in action. You, therefore, live in the Presence of God now. Remind yourself of this as often as necessary until you accept it as naturally as the air you breathe.

Renounce the idea that God is removed from you, that you have to work hard to earn God's grace or to awaken to realization of God. Those erroneous ideas are two of the primary awareness-clouding delusions that keep many people in self-imposed spiritual bondage. Absolutely refuse to deny your divine nature. Do not listen to anyone who tries to convince you that you are anything but a perfect, God-expressing being. Keep your own counsel. Know the truth and live it to the fullest extent possible. It is by living what you know that you learn and grow. Your potential to experience the unfoldment of soul knowledge and to actualize your innate divine qualities and capacities is virtually limitless.

Physical aging is considered normal for human beings and most other forms of life on Planet Earth. While a few simple organisms renew themselves almost endlessly unless their existence is terminated by accident or oppressive environmental factors, and some trees and shrubs live for thousands of years, people and most other biological life forms seem to be programmed to live for only relatively brief durations of time.

Certain insects live but a few days or weeks, and some animals live but a few years while others live for decades. Life expectancy for people has been rapidly increasing during the past century. One hundred years ago, in Europe and America, the life expectancy of a newborn infant was less than 50 years. Today it is closer to 80 or 90, with increasing numbers of men and women living beyond 100. In 1996 there were approximately 40,000 people in America over 100 years of age, and this age-segment of the population is expected to double by 2050. The numbers of older people are also increasing in several European countries. Many who are living longer are also healthy and active, continue to work or to be involved with projects and relationships, and have a keen interest in what is happening in the world.

It is now widely believed that, with a positive mental attitude and a wholesome lifestyle, it is possible to live 120 or more healthy, productive years. Aging alone is not the cause of physical demise. The cause is almost always a malfunction or breakdown of one or more of the body's life-support systems. Accidents account for many physical deaths and, undoubtedly, there are some instances of conscious withdrawal from the body because the soul considers its mission here to have been completed. Too, there are undoubtedly many instances of withdrawal because one feels that physical life is no longer worth living.

There are several theories about what causes aging. One is that genetic programming determines life-span. Another view is that symptoms of aging accumulate because the body doesn't repair and regenerate itself fast enough to keep pace with the damage inflicted by stress, unhealthy living habits, and environmental contamination. Other determining factors are our expectations about how long it is possible to live and the zest for life and sense of meaningful purpose we have.

Genetic programming is obviously influential to a considerable degree. Among insects, fish and other aquatic creatures, and various members of the animal kingdom, individual life spans within a species are fairly predictable. Creatures are born, live, reproduce, play their role in nature, and die, much as most humans do. They don't think about the processes; they just follow the script. We cannot say that the billions of creatures that die every day (I include insects, which, with an estimated 800,000 species, exceed the entire population of other creatures) do so because they think they must. And we cannot say (as I heard one person suggest) that human beings experience death of the body only because they believe it is inevitable; that they see others die and accept the belief that death is normal. However, a fatalistic mental attitude can contribute to apathy and disinterest in living which may influence a person to engage in self-destructive or unhealthy behaviors that hasten the onset of transition. There is considerable evidence to support the idea that one's expectation of healthy, long life can play a decisive role in determining such an outcome.

There is no possibility of physical immortality because the physical universe is an event occurring in time. The universe emerged from the field of primordial nature and will, after several trillion years, return to it. While the substance of which the universe is formed is as eternal as God, its manifestations occur periodically. Souls have come from God into their relationship with the physical realm through levels of cosmic manifestation and dwell in the universe where they can best function because of their degree of enlightenment or where they have a destiny.

Even though we will not live forever in a physical form, we should think in terms of healthy, vital function for as long as we have reasons for being here. For this, it is helpful to renounce beliefs that are restrictive and behaviors which are self-defeating, and to have an understanding of ourselves in relationship to God and the universe. Respond to the following questions:

- Why are you here?

_____

_____

_____

- Why do you want to live long?

_____

_____

_____

• Review your circumstances, relationships, and behaviors. What are you doing to fulfill your purposes?

_____

_____

_____

If you do not know why you are here, ask until the answer is revealed. Insights will surface in your mind and events will unfold in your life to present you with worthwhile opportunities for learning and serving.

If you do not want to live long, ask yourself, "Why not?" Become aware of self-limiting attitudes and feelings that you might have, why you have them, and what you can do to eliminate them. Remove all restrictions from your life.

If your present circumstances, relationships, and behaviors are not supportive of your known purposes, choose supportive circumstances, relationships, and behaviors. Avoid procrastination, laziness, or making excuses for ineffective living.

It is important that you have knowledge (or at least a perception) of worthwhile purposes in life. When you are intent upon fulfilling your worthwhile purposes, all of your lifestyle and behavioral choices will reflect your motivation. When you are not intent, there may be a tendency to be weak-willed and indecisive, to have vague ideas, not to think clearly, or to go along with whatever is happening at the moment even if it is not in your best interest.

When I was a young adult, I knew I was here to know God and share knowledge of God with others. How this

was to be accomplished was not then known, but awareness of my soul destiny was clear. When I was eighteen, I
was fortunate to read Paramahansa Yogananda's book
Autobiography of a Yogi. A few months later, I traveled to
California to meet him, was accepted for discipleship train-
ing, engaged in intensive study, self-analysis, and spiritual practice, and was ordained by him before my twenty-
first birthday. Although at that time I still had much to
learn, in the years that followed I acquired knowledge
and learned to apply it. I am as enthusiastic and purposeful as ever because I know why I am here and what I
am to do—and I am doing it. You, too, can know why you
are here and what you are to do, and do it with excellence
if you sincerely want to. I hope you do.

You Are Already Experiencing Immortality: Now Choose to Consciously *Experience It*

As a ray of the light of God's consciousness, you need
not desire immortality—you *are* immortal. All that is
needed is to choose to consciously experience the freedom
you can have for the accepting. You can be enlightened—
completely knowledgeable about yourself, God, and the
processes of life—while embodied. Then, when your
sojourn in this realm is concluded, you will continue to
experience conscious immortality in subtle and fine realms
until you awaken completely in God.

Contemplate the possibilities before you, rather than
be resigned to a life of ordinary, self-conscious, unaware
existence. All obstacles can be removed, all problems can
be solved, and all inner restrictions can be dissolved. You
need not pretend that you are a victim of circumstances

beyond your control. You need not be at the mercy of painful memories of past unpleasant experiences, beliefs, desires, or actions. You need not be conflicted by thoughts or feelings of guilt, poor self-esteem, or any other idea or feeling. You need not be the effect of karma, planetary influences, environmental conditions, or any other situation. The cosmic forces in the field of nature will be supportive of you when you are living with enlightened understanding and fulfilling your soul destiny.

During the present incarnation you have experienced the soul's superiority over the mind and body. You have made choices. You have experienced the successful outcomes of your intentions and constructive actions. Your body's cells are constantly being replaced. You have a new stomach lining every five days, a new covering of skin every five weeks, and new bones every three months. The atoms of your body have been replaced countless times. You have, therefore, already lived in and expressed through several physical bodies during the years you have been on earth since you were born.

Your body's intelligence can regrow a new liver if two-thirds of it is removed. If a small child's fingertip is severed, it will grow a new one. The body's ability to spontaneously regenerate new limbs and most organs usually ceases before the onset of puberty, but there is the possibility that regenerative powers can be restored. Nerve cells, once believed to be irreplaceable, can often be regenerated. Any part of the body that has been impaired is capable of being restored to function. The intelligence which directed the formation of your body in your mother's womb can direct regenerative processes when encouraged (or allowed) to do so. For instance, a mild electric current administered to broken bones can quicken the healing process. Rest, good nutrition, visualization, and the healing currents of vital force can contribute to rapid healing of the body and its maintenance.

While 120 healthy, functional years is the estimated achievable life-span for most human beings of our present era, there are records of some individuals who have far surpassed this number. In 1963, the Indian saint known as the Shivapuri Baba left his body at the age of 138. He was a lifelong devotee of God and lived very simply. The first 25 years of his adult life were devoted to the study of scriptures and spiritual practice in the seclusion of a forest. Afterward, until age 90, he traveled the world to meet with sincere truth seekers. For the remaining 48 years he lived at his quiet wooded retreat in Nepal.

Another Indian yogi, Sadhu Tapasviji, lived for well over a century and a half. His life was arduous. After raising a family he left home at age 55 to embark on an enlightenment quest, visiting ashrams and pilgrimage sites, alternated by long periods of self-imposed seclusion for the purpose of nurturing superconscious and God-conscious states. During his eighth decade, physically exhausted, he happened to meet a person knowledgeable in an Ayurvedic rejuvenation procedure known as *kaya-kalpa* who offered to assist him. After undergoing a detoxification program, he retired to a closed building which had been specially prepared for his use and remained there for three months. During that time he did not speak. The first several days were spent in deep sleep. When he was rested, he meditated constantly, except for taking his daily meal—which consisted of boiled milk, small portions of nutrition-rich foods, and an herbal compound prescribed for its vitalizing effects.

When he emerged after his three-month retreat, he appeared to be in his mid-fifties. His once scant, white hair was full and black, his skin was radiant, his eyesight was clear, and he had grown new teeth. He later said that his weeks of secluded rest had been beneficial, the cleansing routines and the special foods and herbs had been helpful, but the most influential part of the therapy was the several weeks of meditation and samadhi (superconsciousness) which kept him absorbed in the Infinite. When he was 150 years of age he again underwent the regeneration regimen, and still again a few years later. Finally, in his 168th year, he left his body during meditation.

Not all enlightened souls choose to live long in the body. Some are born to fulfill specific purposes. When their work is done, they return their awareness to astral or causal realms or remove awareness from involvement with all realms and consciously rest in the samadhi (oneness, wholeness) of pure consciousness.

In an ancient Vedic scripture, cleansing procedures for the purpose of liberating the soul's qualities and forces are described:

> The freedom of spiritual mastery can be accomplished by purification of the gross physical, subtle astral, and fine causal bodies (including the mind). It is also possible by God's grace.
>
> Purification of the physical body can easily be accomplished by natural means; purification of the astral body can be accomplished by disciplined cultivation of patience in all circumstances; purification of the fine causal body and of the mind can be accomplished by meditative absorption in Om.

The first verse of chapter four of Patanjali's *Yoga Sutras* provides similar information:

> One may be born with awakened soul abilities. They can also be unfolded by the use of natural substances, the power of mantra, self-discipline, and practice of samadhi (superconsciousness).

Physical cleansing is accomplished by having a clean, natural environment, moderate fasting, eating pure foods, drinking pure water, bathing, enemas when needed, sweating, water and herbal oil cleansing of the nasal passages and sinuses, oil massage, and the use of specific herbs. In some instances, for the advanced rejuvenation regimen, the burnt ashes of certain gemstones and metals (which have been purified by intense heat and ground to an extremely fine powder) are taken with herbs. These are believed to be extremely potent because, unlike food nutrients and herbal essences, they remain in the system for a long time. They must, however, be accurately prescribed, carefully prepared, and precisely used.

For a radical rejuvenation program, the subject must have an understanding of the philosophical principles for which it is practiced, be a proficient meditator, be able to experience isolation for the duration of the program, have no external distractions or sensory stimulation, and avoid reading or talking. A daily routine of gentle hatha yoga practice or simple stretching is helpful to maintaining muscle tone, encouraging blood and lymph circulation, and stimulating glands, organs, and systems of the body. The ideal is to create a "spiritual womb" in which complete rest is assured so that all of the vital forces can be used to regenerate the body's cells, tissues, and organs. One's awareness should be immersed in pure consciousness to the extent possible. Anyone who assists—by providing food and herbal substances, monitoring progress, or rendering therapeutic aid such as massage—should not talk so that the patient can remain in a sustained meditative state. This is a time for complete surrender in the Infinite; not an occasion to engage in idle daydreaming or psychological self-analysis. Awareness should be removed from all distractions, including memories and mental and emotional states.

As a result of deep tissue cleansing, absence of any situation which could cause damage or stress to the systems of the body, transmutation of vital forces, and sustained superconsciousness, the brain secretes a substance referred to as a divine elixir or ambrosia (*amrita*), which further enlivens the physiology and strengthens the immune system.

The Ayurvedic wellness system of northern India at first emphasized foods and herbal substances for physical rejuvenation and health maintenance. The wellness system known as Siddha Medicine, which evolved separately in south India, used regimens similar to Ayurvedic procedures and specialized in the application of purified metal ash. Later, the best of both systems was blended. Agastya, a *siddha* (accomplished) spiritual master who lived in south India several centuries ago, wrote scores of treatises on wellness procedures in Tamil, the language of that region, for the welfare of the general population and for devotees of God who wanted to live long for the purpose of completing their spiritual unfoldment. He, like Mahavatar Babaji in my guru line, is reputed to be a mortal-immortal: an enlightened being who still dwells on the planet in his regenerated physical form.

Purification of the physical body is more rapidly accomplished by living so that entirely *sattvic* (uplifting, illuminating) influences are allowed to be supportive.

Cleansing of the subtle astral body, the soul-covering or sheath of vital forces and the seat of feelings or emotions, is accomplished by disciplined cultivation of equanimity and patience in all circumstances. Regardless of what is observed or experienced, one is advised to be soul-content—not satisfied with challenging situations but inwardly peaceful while solving problems that need to be solved or withdrawing from ones which are not important. It is a matter of learning to be calm, peaceful, and insightful regardless of what is occurring within one's own mind, the immediate environment, or the universe. Perfecting the *yamas* (restraints) and *niyamas* (constructive actions) of yoga is helpful to this end. The restraints are: harmlessness, honesty, truthfulness, conservation and transmutation of vital forces, and renunciation of mental and emotional attachments. The constructive actions are: inner and outer purity, soul-contentment, self-analysis and other practices to ensure psychological health, study of the nature of the soul and God, and surrender of self-consciousness to awaken to superconscious states.

Actualizing patience encourages emotional and spiritual maturity. Patience is demonstrated by peacefully waiting for the unfoldment of desired outcomes without being frustrated or disturbed by mental or emotional conflicts. Because of the soul-mind-body relationship, when there are mental and emotional conflicts or blockages, spiritual growth is usually restricted and physiological functions are disturbed. Psychological unrest contributes to physical discomfort and disharmony, weakens the immune system, interferes with hormonal and biochemical processes, and is often a prelude to accidents.

I know it is not easy for a person with heavy responsibilities and, sometimes, many challenges to be confronted, to quickly master the discipline of patience. Yet, it is important to accomplish it. Philosophical reflection and regular meditation are extremely helpful in cultivating patience. Understanding provides insight into causes and their effects and enables one to "be in the world but not of it." Meditation provides conscious, satisfying experience of wholeness. Also helpful is to learn to flow with life's rhythms and unfolding events, focusing on constructive matters and disregarding, when possible, that which contributes to mental confusion and emotional conflict. Above all, avoid contests with negative people or circumstances. Always choose to think, feel, and do only that which is wholesome and elevating.

"Feed" your mind with valid (truthful) information and constructive ideas by acquiring knowledge from authoritative sources. Monitor your mental and verbal talk and use your powers of intellectual determination to accept only what is true and worthwhile. "Fast" from negative thinking, and from moodiness and other mind-clouding emotional states.

Purification of the astral body is accomplished more quickly when the soul's creative forces (*shakti*) are awakened and flow freely. Soul forces can awaken spontaneously, and they can be encouraged to awaken by sustained aspiration for spiritual growth, prayer, meditation, wholesome living, and mental and spiritual attunement with enlightened people.

The subtle soul sheath is cleansed by merging in Om, the Word or creative energy of God. When meditating, after preliminary procedures have calmed the body and mind, listen to the inner sound. Imagine that it pervades the universe and melt in it. Your mind will be purified, and superconscious influences will flow into deeper layers of your subtle body to enliven it and make it more radiant. Regularly engage in this meditation practice for years. Doing so will take your attention to the Source of everything, to the heart of God.

Sudden illumination of mind can result in immediate cleansing. It is more usual, however, that the mind is cleansed gradually over a period of time. Deep-seated impressions of memories, beliefs, and habits will be organized and disarmed. Their influential force will be weakened and neutralized. In this way, karma is eradicated because of your commitment to spiritual growth and regular meditation practice. Some mental conditionings will have to be confronted and discarded by choice.

You can decide not to let memories of pain and misfortune influence your mind or emotions. You can replace nonuseful or destructive habits with useful, constructive behaviors. You can modify desires and change your course in life by deciding to do so. Your intentional, constructive actions will enable you to master your states of consciousness, mental states, emotional states, behaviors, and how you perceive your world and respond to it.

Purification is accomplished quickly by cultivating devotion to God and renouncing self-consciousness (egoism, the illusional sense of being an entity independent of God) so that your innate urge to have awareness completely restored to wholeness can be efficiently fulfilled. If you are not now Self-realized, it is only because your awareness is clouded or your attention is overly identified with external circumstances. All that is needed is to return your awareness to the clear state.

See and Accept Your Highest Good and Be Responsive to God's Fulfilling Grace

You are in this world, learning more, and becoming proficiently functional because of God's grace. You are becoming more skillfully and effectively involved with the processes of life because of God's grace. You are experiencing authentic spiritual growth because of God's grace. You are awakening from the "dream" of mortality because of God's grace. *Grace is the active expression of impulses originating in the field of divine consciousness contributing to evolutionary unfoldments and spiritual growth.* The actions of grace express from within us from the soul level, and around us because God's Reality is omnipresent.

You did not become involved with the field of nature because you did anything wrong, but because you were meant to do so. Make the most of your opportunity. Don't blame God, circumstances, or yourself for being here. Confront the situation with the knowledge you have; be courageous; grow in understanding and functional ability.

Narrow-minded preoccupation with self-centered interests, dependent emotional attachments, allowing destructive or nonuseful mental conditionings and habits to dominate consciousness and determine behaviors, lack of "will to live," mental confusion, emotional unrest, a perverse mental attitude that causes one to distort information for self-serving purposes, physical discomfort or unwellness, restrictive circumstances of all kinds, and all other limiting conditions are obstacles to Self-realization and Self-actualization. Every obstacle can be removed by right understanding and right living. The radiance of the soul then shines by itself.

By doing what you can to live righteously (correctly, in accord with the causative laws or principles of nature) and to nurture spiritual growth, you will know peace and continue to grow in understanding and grace. Train yourself to be open to and accepting of your highest good in every aspect of your life. You need not agree to any other condition. To do so is to deny the truth of your being—to impose upon yourself limitations of your own creation.

The constructive things you do can improve your circumstances and encourage the unfoldment and self-manifestation of your "inner splendor." Your actions are more effective when performed with clear knowledge of your relationship to God and nature. You are a spiritual being. Live from that understanding.

Be Happy, Healthy, and Prosperous

You are here to let the glorious life of God express through and as you. Do these things:

- *Be happy* – Train yourself to always be inwardly happy regardless of outer circumstances. Circumstances change; you, as a spiritual being, are changeless. Rest in permanent awareness of soul and be happy. You can do it by choice.
- *Be healthy* – Help yourself to total wellness by doing what contributes to it and by letting your inner radi-

ance express freely through your mind and body.

- *Be Prosperous* – Be willing to thrive, flourish, and be successful. If you are not willing to be prosperous, you cannot accomplish your purposes or grow spiritually. Confront the need to be prosperous directly. Do not withhold yourself from participation in life's unfolding processes or deny yourself the good fortune that is available to you. Be prosperous in all ways and bless others with your prosperity consciousness and actions. Your highest good is available.

- *Use Energies and Time Wisely* – Thoughts, emotional states, relationships, and activities impelled by whims serve no useful purpose. Abandon them immediately. Be emotionally mature—responsible and focused on essential matters. You will perceive clearly, function effectively, and fulfill your spiritual destiny.

One should choose as a means of livelihood those activities
which are consistent with *dharma* [virtue, righteousness],
adhere to the path of peace, and engage in studies to acquire
useful knowledge. This is the way to happiness.
– *Charaka Samhita* –

Your Personal Application of
Life-Knowledge Program #5

1. Read this book several times, marking with a pencil or pen the themes that speak directly to you. Write your hopes and dreams and your specific action plans for using your knowledge for highest benefits.

_____

_____

_____

_____

_____

_____

_____

Affirm With Quiet Enthusiasm

Yes! I wholeheartedly agree to be happy, healthy, and prosperous in every way. I demonstrate my choice by the thoughts I think, the actions I perform, and my responsiveness to God's blessing-grace as it reveals itself in timely, supportive ways. Established in the freedom of understanding, I quietly and appropriately share my light with others.

APPENDIX

The Inner World of Colors
Gemstones, Metals, and Mantras

Their Special Qualities and Beneficial
Applications According to Ancient Traditions
and Modern Discoveries

The Inner World of Colors,
Gemstones, Metals, and Mantras

The universe we live in is pervaded by an ocean of electromagnetic radiation. We see only a fraction of the visible electromagnetic spectrum; the larger, invisible portion can be detected and measured by instruments invented for that purpose. All of the various kinds of radiant energy, from long waves to short—from radio waves to TV, FM, infrared, the visible spectrum, ultraviolet, X-rays, and gamma rays—have identical physical properties and can be referred to as light waves.

Light is energy emitted from atoms in tiny bursts called photons which travel in wavy motions. Different kinds of atoms emit different kinds of waves. An electron orbiting the nucleus of an atom is given energy when it receives radiation or collides with a neighboring atom. This influx of energy boosts the electron to a higher orbit. The electron's natural tendency to seek its lowest energy state causes it to drop back down. As the electron falls to its lower level it releases its excess energy as a photon of light. An electron dropping between two given orbits will always produce a photon of one specific wavelength.

The seven wavelengths or colors of visible light we normally see are red, orange, yellow, green, blue, indigo, and violet. The eyes of bees and some other insects are evolved to enable them to see wavelengths that humans cannot see. A light wave with little energy is red. Colors change as the quantity of energy increases. They can be remembered by assigning them the name ROY G. BIV, with

How Light is Produced

An electron orbiting the nucleus of an atom is impacted with energy (*left side of diagram*) when it receives radiation or collides with another atom. The transmitted energy boosts the electron to a higher orbit (*center*). The electron's tendency to seek its lowest energy state causes it to drop down. When falling to its lower level, the electron releases excess energy as a photon of light. An electron dropping between given orbits will always produce a photon of light of one specific wavelength.

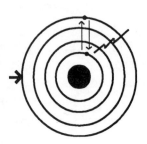

Gamma rays
X-Rays
Ultraviolet
Indigo
Blue
Green
Yellow
Orange
Red
Infrared
Microwaves
TV, FM
Radio waves

THE ELECTROMAGNETIC SPECTRUM

Only wavelengths that produce the colors red to violet are visible to human sight. Red is produced by a low frequency long wave. Violet is produced by a high frequency short wave. Photons traveling at a speed of 860,300 miles a second are measured in angstroms, micrometers, centimeters and meters. All invisible and visible electromagnetic frequencies are light.

each letter representing a color of the visible light spectrum. Light from the Sun is made up of different kinds of waves. The Sun's rays, decomposed when shining through water droplets in the atmosphere, are viewed as a rainbow in the same order of colors that results when sunlight passes through a prism.

Color is not really innate to an object. How light is reflected from an object determines the color we see. When something appears red, for instance, it absorbs all of the colors of light except red. Because black objects absorb all light, no color is reflected. When light is absent, objects cannot be said to be of any color.

Light plays a vital role in nature. Chlorophyll in the cells of green plants converts sunlight to chemical energy and synthesizes organic compounds from inorganic compounds, such as carbohydrates from carbon dioxide and water, accompanied by a release of oxygen: a process known as photosynthesis. What is not so commonly known is that light also directly influences biological forms. Light received through our eyes influences the pituitary gland which regulates the secretions of the endocrine glands and other chemical processes in the body.

Some people who are deprived of sunlight because of staying indoors most of the time or who live in regions where winter months are cloudy and dark, experience mental and emotional depression because of what is called "seasonal affective disorder" (SAD). This condition can usually be remedied by daily exposure to artificial bright light (preferably using full-spectrum light tubes or bulbs when available). Although light entering the eyes directly influences the pituitary gland, the skin of the body can also respond to light.

It is known that the egg production of chickens is increased by extending the hours of light in their environment. In regions of the world that have more hours of daily sunlight, vegetables that grow above the ground are larger than in regions where the hours of sunlight are fewer. Exposure to sunlight (or artificial bright light if sunlight is not available) after a duration of many hours of air travel can reset the body's chemistry and reduce the symptoms of jet-lag: physical tiredness and mental disorientation that often result from east or west long-distance travel through several time zones.

Providing the body with all colors of the spectrum can contribute to our total well-being. There are published anecdotes of individuals who have experienced improvement or healing of arthritis, tiredness, vision problems, and more, as a result of daily exposure to outdoor light. This is most conveniently done by exposure to the Sun's rays for at least one hour every day without the use of eyeglasses. It is not necessary to actually be in direct sunlight because the full spectrum of light is present in shady areas also, but it is important not to wear eyeglasses or contact lenses during this time.

When sunlight is filtered through eyeglasses or through windows of a building or automobile, its varied wavelengths are altered; more so when light is filtered through colored glass. When sunglasses are routinely worn to reduce glare, the tint should be neutral grey. Rose red, green, blue, yellow, or other colors should be avoided because they block the transmission of some of the wavelengths of sunlight while concentrating the color of the eyeglass lenses. Indoor living or work spaces should have windowpanes of clear glass only.

Choosing Colors for
Specific Purposes

Ayurveda considers color to be a subtle form of nutrition for the body's life force, the mind, and the impressions which nourish them. Our body and mind not only absorb colors, they also produce them. The actions of life forces in the body produce colors corresponding to their frequencies and how they are influenced by our mental and emotional states. The colors of the body's aura can reveal prevailing physical and mental states and states of consciousness. Colors can be visualized and projected into one's field of awareness and the physical body for specific purposes. If we feel that we need the influence of certain colors and they are not immediately available in our environment, we can visualize them as being present in the mind or body.

Disharmonious colors can derange mental activity and emotions, and harmonious colors can balance them. Bright colors are stimulating and energizing; dark colors are suppressive. For therapeutic purposes, exposure of the body to lights of prescribed colors can be helpful. Dark blue light, for instance, may be used to heal an infected skin lesion or wound. For general purposes, we can expose ourselves to colors by the clothing we choose to wear and how we choose to paint or decorate our living and work environment.

For overall well-being, we should use *sattvic* colors: white, gold, blue and other colors which affect us harmoniously. Colors can have elevating influences if they are pleasant to live with and make only a mild impression on the senses. *Rajasic* colors are bright, intense, artificial, clashing, and penetrating. Gentle stimulation of *rajas guna* can be provided when desired by the use of yellow, orange, red, and purple. Their excessive use may over-stimulate the mind and senses. Dull, dark, and murky colors are *tamasic* and devoid of energy. They have a dulling effect on the mind and senses.

It is increasingly recognized that full-spectrum light in a work environment promotes cheerfulness and improves efficiency. Thoughtfully chosen decorator colors have similar effects.

White is cool, moist, and nurturing. It has a mild cleansing effect, calms the mind and emotions, and imparts vitality. Excessive use of white can diminish energy and cause a person to become too passive.

Black can have a suppressive influence, although when appropriately used with clothing or decorative objects in harmony with other colors it can reveal a sense of one's dignity and demonstrate originality. Morbid preoccupation with black, or other dark or drab colors, can indicate moodiness, mental depression, or a psychological disorder. Certain shades of dark blue are referred to by some artists as "the blue of madness" because a few famous painters who were believed to be psychotic were fond of using them.

Grey, a combination of white and black, is neutral.

Green is neutral, calming, and moistening. It can be used to neutralize excess mental and emotional "hotness" and balance metabolic processes.

Red stimulates. In milder shades, it can energize and strengthen. In excess, it can provoke anger and a tendency toward violence. It increases *pitta* influences and decreases *vata* and *kapha* influences.

Blue is calming and inspires detachment. It is said to nurture solitude and meditation. Dark or sky blue is cold and dry. Lighter blue, with white, is moistening. It can be used to neutralize hot mental and emotional states. Light blue, white, and gold are good colors for a meditation chapel or for one's private meditation sanctuary. These colors strengthen *sattvic* influences.

Yellow is warm and moistening. It is energizing and nurtures happiness and creativity. If used excessively when *vata* is aggravated, it can nurture behaviors which are superficial and assertive.

Gold harmonizes mental activities and strengthens the heart, circulatory system, glands, and immune system. It nurtures spiritual aspiration.

Orange is warm, energizing, and nurtures intelligence and spiritual awareness.

Brown is stabilizing and neutral.

For strengthening, weakening, or balancing the influences of the three *doshas* as they relate to your basic mind-body constitution, the following recommendations for color usage can be considered.

Warm, moist, soft, and calming colors are advised to balance *vata dosha*. These could be the warm colors of gold, red, orange, and yellow along with moist and calm colors such as white or light shades of blue or green. Bright colors may aggravate or strengthen *vata* characteristics; strong colors may be too stimulating; grey, black, and murky brown may be devitalizing, although in moderation they may have a stabilizing influence.

Cool, mild, and calming colors such as white, green, and blue are advised to balance *pitta dosha*. Colors that are hot and stimulating should be used only infrequently.

Mild shades of color are best, as bright colors of all kinds can be disturbing.

Warm, dry, and mildly stimulating colors such as red, orange, yellow, and gold are advised for balancing *kapha dosha*. Excessive use of white or pastel blues and greens should be avoided. Brighter colors are better.

Almost everyone has a mixture of *dosha* influences in their mind-body constitution and suitable colors can be chosen accordingly.

The Inner World of Gemstones

The color of gemstones is the basis for using them for balancing physical and mental energies. They are usually worn in a ring on a finger or as a pendant on a chain around the neck. For beneficial purposes, the ring or pendant is open at the back so the stone can touch the skin. It is not only our sight perception of the color of the gemstones that is influential—ions radiated by them are said to be received through the skin to influence the atoms of our bodies. The Greek word *ion* means "something that goes." An ion is an atom or group of atoms, originally neutral, that has acquired an electric charge by gaining or losing electrons. Electromagnetic forces are also believed to radiate from gemstones to influence body chemistry and the various aspects of *prana* flowing through the *prana* channels (*nadis*).

Paramahansa Yogananda's guru, Sri Yukteswar, taught that electric and magnetic radiations circulating in the universe can beneficially and adversely affect body and mind. He explained that ancient seers discovered that pure metals and certain gemstones worn against the skin could be helpful in counteracting the adverse effects of these influences. Sri Yukteswar taught that all parts of creation are linked together and interchange their influences. In our human aspect, we have to contend with two kinds of forces—those in our body-mind constitution, caused by the mixed actions of earth, water, fire, air, and ethereal elements; and those of outer nature. "There are certain mechanical features in the law of karma (causation)," he said, "that can be skillfully adjusted if one has the knowledge to do so."

Although Paramahansaji seldom publicly discussed this subject, he sometimes privately advised certain individuals to obtain and wear a bracelet or bangle made of gold, silver, and copper wires twisted together. Gold is said to be heating to the system, silver is cooling, and copper is purifying. This combination of pure metals is prescribed for balancing and strengthening the body's electromagnetic field. As with gemstones, metal arm bangles used for remedial purposes or for maintaining balance of the body's systems, are of prescribed weight.

Gemstones and metals may be recommended as supplemental aids to balancing the influences of the three *doshas* along with other Ayurvedic regimens, or prescribed for astrological purposes. Gemstones should be without flaws and at least two carats in weight. Less expensive gemstones, when substituted, can be of heavier carat weight as it is believed that their influence is not as great. I do not know whether this is true or whether the *belief* in the potency of gemstones which are considered to be precious because of their rarity and durability is the reason for their being recommended. The crystal structure of gemstones is also believed to be a factor in their capacity to emanate radiations.

Only when certain constituent elements of the earth's inner magma (molten matter which when cooled becomes igneous or fire-formed rock) combine under great pressure in precise proportions and cool and solidify at a certain rate, are crystals produced that are radiant and durable enough to be chosen as gemstones. Diamonds, for instance, made of tightly bonded carbon atoms, are believed to have been formed approximately 100 miles below the surface of the earth in the upper part of the mantle, the 1,800-mile thick region between the molten outer core and the rocky crust. Successful endeavors to produce synthetic diamonds indicate that temperatures slightly above 2,700 degrees Fahrenheit (1482 degrees Celsius) and pressures of 975,000 pounds per square inch are needed to cause carbon to form as diamond crystals. These are then forced to the earth's surface by immense pressure caused by the movements of the earth's crust and volcanic eruptions.

Igneous rock emerging on the surface of the planet is eventually worn down by water, wind, ice, and chemicals in the atmosphere. Fragments are carried away by wind, moving water, and gravity, and settle as sediment on plains, on riverbeds, and at the bottom of the seas. Under the weight of further accumulated debris, the fragments are compacted to form sedimentary rock, including sandstone, limestone, and shale. Before being worn down, igneous rock cools into rock such as granite. At deeper levels, trace elements of molten rock can become concentrated, producing magma rich in water, rare elements, and gases. The water slows the solidification process, and crystal deposits can occur which may contain topaz, tourmaline, aquamarine, and garnet.

When gem crystal-bearing rocks are dispersed by nature's forces and actions, hard gemstones are carried to stream beds. Some gemstones, such as turquoise and opal, form in sedimentary rock as seeping groundwater collects and deposits traces of silica for opal and minerals for turquoise.

Gemstones are also produced in metamorphic rock, which is produced when volcanic activity changes the character of igneous rock. Trace minerals may then be freed to concentrate as gems such as garnet and sapphire. Aluminum oxide or corundum is called ruby when red, and sapphire when blue or other colors.

When white light passes freely through a gemstone it is colorless. The colors of zircons and smoky quartz are caused by light reflecting from their unique crystal structures. Most colors of gemstones are due to the presence of small quantities of metals: mainly iron, chrome, cobalt, copper, manganese, nickel, and vanadium which absorb certain wavelengths of white light.

A gemstone's crystal structure is determined by the order of arrangement of its atoms. The strength of the bonds of its atoms determines a crystal's hardness. Hardness is measured as the amount of resistance to scratching. In 1812, Friedrich Mohs, a German scientist, devised a system for measuring gemstone hardness which is still used. On the Mohs' scale of 1 to 10, starting with talc as the softest mineral, gypsum is 2, calcite 3, fluorite 4, apatite 5, orthoclase 6, quartz (citrine, amethyst, smoky quartz and other quartz gemstones) 7, topaz 8, corundum (rubies and sapphires) 9, and diamond 10. Substances with higher numbers can scratch those with lower numbers. Substances that can scratch the lower numbered ones but not those of the next higher number are numbered between them. An example is emerald (belonging to the beryl group) which has a hardness of 7.5. Quartz, including sand and particles of dust in the air, will scratch all gemstone substances with a number lower than 7. Higher numbered gemstones, which include topaz, ruby, sapphire, and diamond are not scratched by quartz and are considered among the more precious gemstones because of their brightness and durability. The hardness represented by the Mohs' scale is not uniform. There is a greater difference in hardness between diamond and corundum (ruby and sapphire) than between corundum and talc.

Hard gemstones may also be brittle, and easily chipped or shattered. Gemstones that are both hard and tough are best suited for mounting in rings. Diamond, ruby, and sapphire are in this category. Zircon, topaz, emerald, aquamarine, and opal are subject to chipping and breakage. When not being worn, gemstones should be stored separately to avoid being scratched or damaged.

Gemstones are usually designated by carat weight. The name *carat* may be derived from the seed (*kuara*) of the African coraltree or from the kernel (Greek *kertion*) of the carob bean used by traders to measure gemstone weights centuries ago. (The carat weight of gems should not be confused with the word carat (karat) used by goldsmiths to indicate the gold content of an item of manufactured jewelry, which is usually a mixture of gold and copper or some other metal to make it more durable.) For gemstones, one carat equals one fifth of a gram. Divisions of carat weight are called points. Thus, a 100 point stone is one carat, and a 50 point stone is a half carat. Because the specific gravity (the ratio of weight of an equal vol-

ume of water) of gemstones varies, different kinds of gemstones of identical carat weight will not be the same size.
For instance, ruby or sapphire have a higher specific gravity than diamond or emerald and are slightly smaller than
a diamond of equal carat weight.

Much of the attractiveness of some faceted gemstones
is their iridescence because of their optical qualities.

Luster is actually light produced and emitted from
within the gemstone. The impact of external light causes
electrons of the chemical atoms to temporarily move to a
higher orbit then drop back to their original ones, releas-
ing energy as light that glows from within the stone. The
most appealing luster is adamantine (Greek, diamond-
like, bright and clear); the most common is vitreous or
glass-like. Less common are fatty, metallic, pearly, silky,
and waxy lusters. Stones with little or no luster are described as dull or lifeless.

The *refractive index* of a gemstone is determined by
comparing the speed of light in air to its speed when pass-
ing through gemstone crystals. A decrease in the velocity
of light in a stone causes a deviation of the light rays so
that the emergence of reflected light varies, causing a spar-
kling effect. Most gemstones, because of their crystal structure, are doubly refractive.

Color *dispersion* is caused by white light splitting into
its spectral colors. Colorless diamonds of good quality are
noted for their display of dispersed light or "fire."

The *absorption spectra* enables a jeweler to identify
gemstones by determining how light waves pass through
them. This is particularly useful in examining stones of
similar color and specific gravity.

Pleochroism is the property some gem crystals have

of exhibiting two or more colors when viewed from different directions. This is caused by the differing absorption of light of doubly refractive crystals.

Asterism is the effect of light rays forming a star (Greek *aster*) when the rays meet in one point in rounded, smoothly polished stones.

Luminescence (Latin *light*) is the definition for the emission of visible light from a gemstone because of a physical or chemical reaction. The luminescence under ultraviolet light is called fluorescence, caused by metal impurities in the stone.

Several kinds of synthetic gemstones can be produced, which visually appear to be identical to their nature-formed counterparts. While their color may be good, their crystal structure may not be the same as the natural stones and their use is not recommended for remedial or life-enhancing purposes.

Gemstones and metals may be prescribed based on one's astrological chart or according to the Ayurvedic theory of the three *doshas*. Astronomy is the study of planetary movements. The study of planetary relationships and interplanetary magnetism and its influences is called astrology. In ancient (and modern) India this speciality is called *Jyotish*: the study and application of light. Vedic astrology, sometimes called Hindu astrology, is based on the Sidereal zodiac of fixed stars and constellations. Western astrology is based on the Tropical zodiac calculated according to the orientation of our planet to the Sun. The astrological information presented here is based on Jyotish, the Vedic system, which is compatible with the philosophical views of Ayurveda.

Vedic astrological texts refer to only seven planets

because Pluto and Neptune were not discovered until centuries after the calculations for Vedic astrology were formulated. Besides the Sun, Moon (which is considered to be a planet for the purposes of astrological determinations), Mars, Venus, Mercury, Saturn, and Jupiter, the north and south nodes of the Moon are considered as "shadow planets" because of their influences on Planet Earth's magnetic field.

The north node of the Moon, or Dragon's head, is given the Sanskrit name Rahu. The south node of the Moon, the Dragon's tail, is given the name Ketu. Astronomically, the two lunar nodes represent points at which the Moon's orbit crosses the ecliptic, the celestial equator. These are places at which the Moon crosses the point of the Sun's orbit where eclipses can occur. The lunar nodes indicate to an astrologer the times when solar and lunar forces obstruct or cancel each other.

The ascending node, Rahu, is the point at which the Moon crosses the ecliptic to the north; the descending node, Ketu, is where it crosses to the south. The influence of the north node is said to be expanding and externalizing but not always in constructive ways. The influence of the south node is contracting and internalizing.

To have a horoscope accurately determined and interpreted in a meaningful way by a competent astrologer, we need to provide the exact time and location of birth. A competent astrologer must be well-trained in the art of preparing a horoscope, a wise philosopher, and spiritually aware enough to be able to interpret the chart on all levels in relationship to the client's state of consciousness and karmic condition. Otherwise, the information given to the client may be erroneous, misleading, or superficial.

Our horoscope does not proclaim an event that impacted us at birth; it merely reveals the degree of soul unfoldment and the karmic condition when we came into this world. Our mental and emotional conditionings—our influential memories, desires, habits, tendencies, beliefs, and illusions—comprise our karmic condition which can be known, overcome, or transcended. According to the philosophical teachings of Vedic seers, conception and birth occur when one's karmic condition is in accord with those incidents. As spiritual beings, we only identify with and express through the body and mind. Insight into this process can enable us to be dispassionately objective about our relationship with the universe and motivate us to aspire to awaken to complete understanding that liberates our consciousness.

The less spiritually aware we are, the more we are inclined to be at the mercy of our karmic condition and of external causes. The more spiritually aware we are, the more we are enabled to discern the internal causes of problems and weaken, modify, or eliminate them, and to understand, work with, or transcend external influences. The ideal is to cease being a victim of causative influences of any kind, and to flow with the rhythms of life to fulfill soul destiny.

A person who has a failure-attitude will almost invariably choose to dramatize a victim role in relationship to circumstances by passively reacting to causative influences, clinging to erroneous beliefs and opinions, remaining habit-bound, repeating self-defeating behaviors, refusing to learn and to grow, and asserting that circumstances beyond their control are compelling.

A person who has a success-attitude will choose to be

self-responsible, desire to grow to emotional and spiritual maturity, and learn to live in harmony with the Power that enlivens and nurtures the universe.

Choosing and Using Gemstones and Metals for Life-Enhancing Purposes

These descriptions are for gemstones and metals commonly recommended by practitioners of Ayurveda and Jyotish. Information is provided for using this approach to restore and maintain balanced *dosha* influences and for astrological purposes. Anyone can use gems and metals for balancing *dosha* influences. For astrological purposes, the wise counsel of a competent Vedic astrologer is usually needed.

Diamond (Greek *adamus*, unconquerable, hard)
Color: Colorless, yellow, brown, green, blue, red
Mohs' Hardness: 10
Specific Gravity: 3.47–3.55
Crystal System: Isometric (cubic)
Chemical Composition: C, crystallized carbon
Transparency: Transparent
Double Refraction: None
Dispersion: 0.044
Pleochroism: None

Widely used for personal adornment for centuries, the scratch resistance of diamond is 240 times greater than that of corundum (ruby and sapphire).

Colorless diamond is worn to decrease *vata* and *pitta* influences and may mildly increase *kapha*. It is said to strengthen the reproductive system. Yellow gold may be mildly heating to the body's systems; silver is cooling.

Of the less expensive gemstones, colorless sapphire or zircon of good quality may be substituted.

For general astrological purposes, diamond may be worn when Venus influence is weak. Some symptoms of weak Venus influence may be lack of refinement, affection, or sensitivity. There may be weakness of kidneys and of the reproductive system and bones. Energy may be low, the immune system may be weak, and one may be prone to urinary tract infections. Diamond is not recommended if one has a strong sex drive or a compelling need for comfort and affluence. If these drives are deficient, diamond may be recommended.

A diamond of at least one carat, set in yellow or white gold, may be first worn on a Friday when the Moon is waxing, preferably when Venus is exalted. The Sanskrit mantra for Venus influence is *Om Shukraya Namaha*.

Ruby (Latin *rubeu*s, red)
Color: Red
Mohs' Hardness: 9
Specific Gravity: 3.97–4.05
Crystal System: Hexagonal
Chemical Composition: Al_2O_3 aluminium oxide
Transparency: Opaque, translucent, transparent
Refractive Index: 1.766–1.774
Double Refraction: 0.008
Dispersion: 0.018
Pleochroism: Strong; yellow-red, deep ruby red

Until ruby and sapphire were recognized as belonging to the corundum gemstone group, red spinel and garnet were also designated as ruby.

Ruby is used to strengthen the heart, stimulate circulation, improve digestive powers, and increase energy. It increases *pitta* and decreases *vata* and *kapha* influences.

Red garnet or any other less expensive red gemstone of good quality may be substituted.

For general astrological purposes ruby may be worn when Sun influence is weak. Some symptoms of weak Sun influence are lack of self-confidence, self-respect, and strength of will. One may be dependent upon others (or externals) for a sense of identity. There may be low energy, anemia, weak digestive powers, poor appetite, weak or slow pulse, weak heart, poor circulation, arthritis, bone weakness, or poor eyesight.

Ruby (or other dark red gemstones) are not advised if one suffers from fever, bleeding, ulcers, hypertension, or infectious diseases, or if an egocentric drive for power and desire to dominate is excessive.

A ruby of at least two carats, set in yellow gold, may be first worn at sunrise on a Sunday, preferably when the Sun is in its own sign or is exalted. The Sanskrit mantra for Sun influence is *Om Suryaya Namaha.*

Sapphire (Greek word for blue)
Color: Blue
Mohs' Hardness: 9
Specific Gravity: 3.99–4.00
Crystal System: Hexagonal
Chemical Composition: Al_2O_3 aluminum oxide
Transparency: Transparent, opaque
Refractive Index: 1.766–1.774
Double Refraction: 0.008
Dispersion: 0.018
Pleochroism: Definite; dark blue, green-blue

The word sapphire is used to designate blue corundum. Other colors of this gemstone are designated by name: yellow sapphire, orange-pink sapphire called *padparadschah* (Sinhalese for "lotus flower"), green sapphire, purple sapphire, and ruby for red sapphire.

Blue sapphire may be used to provide positive energies, strengthen bones, calm nerves and emotions, and promote an attitude of detachment. It is recommended to be worn in a gold setting for *vata* and *kapha* mind-body constitutions or in silver for *pitta*.

For general astrological purposes blue sapphire may be worn when Saturn influence is weak. Some symptoms of weak Saturn influence may be tremors, inability to manage stress, and lack of mental and emotional calm. There may be poor vitality, bone and nerve weakness, a tendency to be constipated, and slow renewal of tissues.

A blue sapphire of at least two carats, set in yellow gold, may be first worn on a Saturday when the Moon is waxing, preferably when Saturn influences are already beneficially aspected. The Sanskrit mantra for Saturn influence is *Om Shanaischaraya Namaha*.

Yellow Sapphire
Color: Rich yellow to pale yellow, or golden
Mohs' Hardness: 9
Specific Gravity: 3.99–4.00
Crystal System: Hexagonal
Chemical Composition: Al_2O_3 aluminium oxide
Transparency: Transparent, opaque
Refractive Index: 1.766–1.774
Double Refraction: 0.008
Dispersion: 0.018
Pleochroism: Weak; yellow, light yellow

Yellow sapphire is considered to be the best gemstone for promoting overall health. It beneficially influences the endocrine glands and increases the accumulation of refined energy (*ojas*). It has a balancing effect on all three *doshas* and is helpful in decreasing excessive *vata* influences. It is usually worn in a gold setting.

Yellow quartz (citrine) or any other less expensive yellow or golden gemstone (such as yellow or golden beryl or chrysoberyl) of good quality may be substituted.

For general astrological purposes yellow sapphire may be worn when Jupiter influence is weak. Some symptoms of weak Jupiter influence may be diminished joyfulness and enthusiasm, weak will, and lack of faith. There may be moodiness, pessimism, anxiety, self-pity, and lack of compassion. There may be difficulties with material and financial matters. One may have a weak immune system and low vitality. These symptoms are similar to those that indicate a too strong Saturn influence.

A yellow sapphire of at least two carats, set in yellow gold, may be first worn on a Thursday morning when the Moon is waxing and when Jupiter is exalted, is in its own sign, or when in an angle to the Moon. The Sanskrit mantra for Jupiter influence is *Om Brihaspatyaye Namaha.*

Emerald (Greek *Smaragdos*, "green stone")
Color: Green
Mohs' Hardness: 7.5–8
Specific Gravity: 2.67–2.78
Crystal System: Hexagonal
Chemical Composition: $Al_2Be_3(Si_6O_{18})$
    aluminum beryllium silicate
Transparency: Transparent to opaque
Refractive Index: 1.576–1.582
Double Refraction: 0.006
Dispersion: 0.014
Pleochroism: Definite; green, blue-green to yellow-green

Emerald is used to calm the mind and nervous system and improve intellectual powers. It harmonizes *vata* influences, decreases *pitta*, and may mildly increase *kapha*. It may be prescribed for certain degenerative diseases. Individuals with *vata* or *kapha* mind-body constitutions may wear emerald in a gold setting. For *pitta* characteristics, a silver setting is recommended.

Green tourmaline or any other less expensive dark green stone of good quality may be substituted.

For general astrological purposes emerald may be worn when Mercury influence is weak. Some symptoms of weak Mercury influence may be poor communication skills, poor memory, emotional immaturity, addictions, dependencies, intellectual dullness, irrational thinking, and excessive daydreaming. One may also experience weakness of the nervous system, emotional pain, anxiety, insomnia, and allergies.

An emerald of at least two carats, set in yellow gold, can first be worn on a Wednesday, when the Moon is waxing and Mercury is exalted, is in its own sign, or is well-aspected. The Sanskrit mantra for Mercury influence is *Om Budhaya Namaha.*

Pearl (The name is perhaps derived from Latin *perna*, a type
    of shell; or *sphareula*, because of its spherical shape)
Color: White, silver, cream, golden, pink, green, blue, black
Mohs' Hardness: 3–4
Specific Gravity: 2.60–2.78
Crystal System: Microcrystalline
Chemical Composition: 84–92% calcium carbonate,
    4–13% organic substances, 3–4% water
Transparency: Translucent to opaque
Double Refraction: Weak or none

Pearls are not true gemstones. They are formed of calcium carbonate in shells of molluscs, usually oysters. White pearls are usually recommended by Ayurvedic or Jyotish practitioners to beneficially influence body fluids, nourish tissues and nerves, calm the emotions, and strengthen the female reproductive system. Pearl increases *kapha* and decreases *vata* and *pitta*. A single pearl may be worn in a silver setting on the left hand, or a necklace of pearls may be worn.

A less expensive substitute is cultured pearl. Moonstone is also sometimes substituted.

For general astrological purposes pearl can be worn when Moon influence is weak. Some symptoms of weak Moon influence are emotional instability, anxiety, fear of intimacy, and light-mindedness and disorientation. Other symptoms may be anemia, diminished body fluids, dry skin, constipation, weak lungs and kidneys, and low body weight. Women may have menstrual problems or have difficulty conceiving a child.

Pearl is usually not recommended if one is suffering from obesity, edema (water retention), congestion, excessive mucus discharge, or if one is too emotional, sentimental, greedy, or possessive.

A pearl of at least two carats, set in silver, may be first worn on a Monday when the Moon is waxing or is full and when other aspects are supportive. The Sanskrit mantra for Moon influence is *Om Somaya Namaha*.

Red Coral
Color: Red
Mohs' Hardness: 3–4
Specific Gravity: 2.6–2.7
Crystal System: Hexagonal; microcrystalline

Chemical Composition: $CaCO_3$ calcium carbonate
   plus magnesia and organic substances
Transparency: Opaque
Refractive Index: 1.486–1.658
Double Refraction: –0.172

Coral reefs and atolls are formed from calcified skeletons of tiny polyps which secrete a calcite substance. Coral can be red, pink, white, black, or blue. Red coral is generally used for ayurvedic and astrological purposes.

It is said to improve the quality of blood and strengthen the reproductive system (especially of men). It harmonizes *pitta*, decreases *vata*, and may increase *kapha* if the coral piece is too large and one already has a strong *kapha dosha* constitution. It is usually recommended to be worn in a silver setting on the right hand, although it is often worn as a pendant. Because red coral is inexpensive, no substitute is recommended.

For general astrological purposes red coral may be worn when Mars influence is weak. Some symptoms of weak Mars influence may be lack of energy and motivation, fearfulness, passivity, and a tendency to be victimized. Other symptoms may be a weak immune system, diminished appetite and poor digestion and assimilation, muscle weakness, slow healing of injuries, and anemia.

Red coral is usually not recommended if one has a high fever, infection, ulcers, or symptoms of excessive *pitta dosha* influences.

Red coral of at least two carats, set in yellow gold, may be first worn on a Tuesday when the Moon is waxing, preferably when Mars is exalted or well-aspected. The Sanskrit mantra for Mars is *Om Kujaya Namaha*.

Hessonite Garnet (Gomed)
Color: Copper-brown (cinnamon color), golden
Mohs' Hardness: 7–7.5
Specific Gravity: 3.60–3.68
Chemical Composition: $Ca_3Al_2(SiO_4)_3$
    calcium aluminum silicate.
Transparency: Transparent, translucent
Refractive Index: 1.738–1.745
Dispersion: 0.027

The energy of hessonite garnet is neutral and, like yellow sapphire, balances all three *doshas*. It is said to calm the nerves.

For general astrological purposes hessonite garnet may be worn when the influences of Rahu (the north lunar node) need to be regulated. Some symptoms of this condition may be fear, anxiety, hallucinations, drug dependency, moodiness, fantasies, clouded awareness, and unclear perceptions (illusions). Symptoms may be immune system weakness, nervousness, insomnia, diminished control of body functions, and mental disorders.

The gemstone, of at least three carats set in silver or gold, may be first worn on a Saturday when the Moon is waxing, or on the day of the planetary ruler of the horoscope. The Sanskrit mantra for Rahu is *Om Rahava Namaha*.

Cat's Eye (belonging to the *chrysoberyl*, Greek for gold)
    group of gemstones
Color: Golden yellow, green-yellow, brown
Mohs' Hardness: 8.5
Specific Gravity: 3.70–3.72
Crystal System: Orthorhombic
Chemical Composition: $Al2(BeO4)$
    beryllium aluminum oxide

Transparency: Transparent, opaque
Refractive Index: 1.744–1.755
Double Refraction: +0.011
Dispersion: 0.015
Pleochroism: Very weak; reddish-yellow,
    yellow, light green, green

Chrysoberyl may be transparent and suitable for faceting or it may be opaque and prepared in a rounded and polished cabochon-cut. A rare kind of chrysoberyl is the gemstone called alexandrite, with internal characteristics that cause it to appear green in normal daylight and red under incandescent light.

A cabochon-cut (rounded and polished) opaque chrysoberyl gemstone with fine, parallel inclusions that produce a silver-white line that is observed as a moving light ray is referred to as cat's eye.

When worn, cat's eye increases *pitta* and decreases *vata* and *kapha*. It is used to stimulate mental energies and strengthen the nervous system.

For general astrological purposes cat's eye can be worn when the influences of Ketu (the south lunar node) need to be regulated. Some symptoms of this condition may be lack of self-confidence, poor concentration, and weak powers of intellectual discernment. One may have poor eyesight, feel restricted by circumstances, may be prone to violence and to being injured, and may be attached to memories of past misfortune. Other symptoms may be weak digestive powers, poor circulation, bleeding disorders, and problems with muscles and nerves.

This gemstone is not recommended if one is suffering from acute bleeding, high fever, headaches, infections, or other symptoms of excessive *pitta* influences.

A cat's eye of least three carats, set in gold, can be first worn on a Saturday when the Moon is waxing and when Ketu is favorably aspected. The Sanskrit mantra for Ketu is *Om Ketave Namaha.*

For general purposes, gemstones or metals can be selected and used at any time. For astrological purposes, if possible, gemstones should be set in the ring or pendant by a jeweler when the Moon is waxing and the stone's planet is favorably aspected. Before the item is first worn, it can be cleaned and placed on the altar in your personal meditation sanctuary or placed before a picture of a saint whom you revere. If Sanskrit mantras are to be chanted during your private consecration ritual, they should be learned ahead of time and correctly pronounced. If mantras are not used, surrendered prayer and faith in God will be sufficient. When first wearing the item, open your mind and heart (your innermost being) to God. By doing this, it becomes a talisman: special or meaningful to you apart from its possible practical usefulness because you have consecrated and blessed it, and because it can remind you that you are willing to be receptive and responsive to the nurturing forces of the universe.

If you choose to experiment with these processes, do so with discernment. Avoid superstitious beliefs and performance of actions because of faith in magic or chance. Your primary reliance should be upon the application of your knowledge of nature's laws, your ability to live effectively, and God's grace. While gemstone and metal influences may be beneficial if skillfully prescribed and utilized, they are of secondary value.

I salute the supreme teacher, the truth, whose
nature is bliss; who is the giver of the highest
happiness; who is pure wisdom; who is beyond
all qualities and infinite like the sky; who is beyond
words; who is one and eternal, pure and still; who
is beyond all change and phenomena and who is the
silent witness to all our thoughts and emotions.
I salute truth, the supreme teacher.
— Ancient Vedic Hymn —

Bibliography

Charaka. *Charaka Samhita*. Chowkhamba Sanskrit Series, Varanasi (India).

Frawley, David. *The Astrology of the Seers*. Passage Press, Morson Publishing, Salt Lake City, UT.

Frawley, David. *Ayurvedic Healing: A Comprehensive Guide*. Passage Press, Morson Publishing, Salt Lake City, UT.

Davis, Roy Eugene. *Life Surrendered in God* (commentary on Patanjali's Yoga Sutras). CSA Press, Lakemont, GA.

Davis, Roy Eugene. *The Eternal Way: The Inner Meaning of the Bhagavad Gita*. CSA Press, Lakemont, GA.

Lad, Vasant. *Ayurveda: The Science of Self-Healing*. Lotus Press. The Ayurvedic Institute, Albuquerque, NM.

Lederman, Leon M. and Schramm, David N. *From Quarks to the Cosmos*. Scientific American Library, W. H. Freeman and Company, New York, NY.

National Geographic Book Service. *The Incredible Machine*. An examination of the human body and its systems. National Geographic Society, Washington, D.C.

Schumann, Walter. *Gemstones of the World*. Sterling Publishing Company, New York, NY.

Sushruta. *Sushruta Samhita*. Chowkhamba Sanskrit Series, Varanasi (India).

Thakkur, Chandrashekhar G. *Ayurveda: The Indian Art of Medicine*. ASI Publishers, New York, NY.

The Editors of Time-Life Books. *The Visible Universe*. Time-Life Books, Alexandria, VA.

Tyberg, Judith. *The Language of the Gods*. Kalakshetra Publications, Thiruvanmiyur, Madras (India).

Yogananda, Paramahansa. *Autobiography of a Yogi*. Self-Realization Fellowship, Los Angeles, CA.

Walford, Roy L. and Walford, Lisa. *The Anti-Aging Plan*. Four Walls Eight Windows, New York, NY.

CENTER FOR SPIRITUAL AWARENESS
is an international enlightenment movement with offices
and a meditation retreat center on a secluded eleven acre site
in the mountain region of northeast Georgia. Retreats are
offered here several times annually and public meetings and
seminars are presented in major cities of North America and
some other countries. *Truth Journal* magazine, printed
lessons, and books comprise the literature outreach.
CSA Press is the book publishing department.
A free information packet may be requested.

Center for Spiritual Awareness
Lake Rabun Road, Post Office Box 7
Lakemont, Georgia 30552-0007
Telephone (706) 782-4723   Fax (706) 782-4560